RESUSCITATION RULES

© BMJ Books 1999
BMJ Books is an imprint of the BMJ Publishing Group

First published in 1999
by BMJ Books, BMA House, Tavistock Square,
London WC1H 9JR
www.bmjbooks.com

British Library Cataloguing in Publication Data

A catalogue record for this book is available from the
British Library

ISBN 0-7279-1371-9

Also in this series:
Trauma Rules
Tim Hodgetts, Stephen Deane, Keith Gunning

Resuscitation Rules

Tim Hodgetts

*Consultant and Specialty Adviser in Accident and
Emergency Medicine to the Defence Medical Services, and
Visiting Professor of Emergency Medicine and Trauma,
University of Surrey*

Frimley Park Hospital, Camberley, Surrey

and

Nick Castle

Resuscitation Training Officer

Frimley Park Hospital, Camberley, Surrey

Contents

Medical emergencies

Paediatric resuscitation

Contributors

The following are acknowledged for submitting ideas for rules for this book:

Dr Andrew Brett, Specialist Registrar in Accident and Emergency, Leighton Hospital, Crewe

Major Ian Greaves, Consultant in Accident and Emergency Medicine, Peterborough and District General Hospital

Dr Fiona Jewkes, Consultant Paediatric Nephrologist, University Hospital of Wales

Dr Ian Maconochie, Senior Registrar in Paediatrics, St Mary's Hospital, London

Foreword

Resuscitation Rules is the second in a series of *aide mémoires* which are designed to make learning fun, while providing an easily remembered rule in a crisis. This book combines a systematic, evidence-based approach to resuscitation of the seriously ill patient, with a novel series of rules to trigger the memory.

The reason and the exceptions accompany each rule. Where appropriate, an illustration highlighting a key aspect of a rule is included.

It is hoped that these resuscitation rules will be valuable to all those involved in the education of professionals who deliver emergency care both pre-hospital, and in-hospital.

Readers are encouraged to submit their own resuscitation rules for a future edition. All contributors will be acknowledged. Details of how to submit your rules can be found inside the rear cover.

Tim Hodgetts
Nick Castle

Preface

Airway, breathing, and circulation are the pre-requisites of life and the cornerstone to successful resuscitation.

Resuscitation Rules concentrates on this systematic approach and provides a discussion of practical issues and pitfalls in the management of the critically ill. A companion book, *Trauma Rules*, follows the same approach for the management of the seriously injured.

Cardiorespiratory arrest is the final common pathway for all critical illness. The only measures that improve long-term survival are early basic life support and early defibrillation, and this is reflected in the balance of this book. Where guidelines are referred to, the 1998 European Resuscitation Council (ERC) recommendations on basic and advanced life support are regarded as the standard.[1,2]

But is this emphasis on resuscitation misguided? Maximal clinical effort should be directed towards *preventing* rather than treating cardiorespiratory arrest. This has been recognised as important when treating the critically ill child, as cardiac arrest is invariably secondary to a period of prolonged hypoxia and responds poorly to resuscitative measures.[3] It is also recognised by the development of adult peri-arrest arrhythmia protocols, designed to treat cardiac rhythms that herald cardiac arrest or its recurrence.[4]

Despite this awareness of critically ill children, a staggering deficiency in the care of adult patients prior to admission to an intensive care unit has been identified. Fifty-four of 100 patients received

[1] Advanced Life Support Working Group of the European Resuscitation Council. The 1998 European Resuscitation Council guidelines for adult advanced life support. *BMJ* 1998;**316**:1863–9.
[2] Basic Life Support Working Group of the European Resuscitation Council. The 1998 European Resuscitation Council guidelines for adult single rescuer basic life support. *BMJ* 1998;**316**:1870–6.
[3] Advanced Life Support Group. *Advanced Paediatric Life Support*, 2nd edn. London: BMJ Publishing Group, 1997.
[4] Chamberlain D. Periarrest arrhythmias. *Br J Anaesth* 1997;**79**:198–202.

"suboptimal care" in relation to ABC management.[5] The mortality in this group was 48%, almost twice that of the patients who had been managed "optimally". The problems highlighted were failures of organisation, a lack of clinical knowledge, a failure to appreciate clinical urgency (and therefore late referrals to the intensive care unit), a lack of supervision, and a failure to seek advice.

Suggested opportunities for improving the pre-arrest management of the critically ill have included increasing the seniority of the doctors assessing and treating the patients. While this is attractive, the supporting evidence is not convincing and an increase of consultant-assessed major trauma victims by 28% to 70% had no effect on mortality in a regional trauma centre in the UK.[6]

An alternative is to accept that cardiac arrest is preceded by premonitory symptoms and signs, and to provide hospital-based *medical emergency teams* with specific activation criteria (to include physiological and biochemical parameters, and high risk conditions).[7] Such a team would function in a similar manner to the *trauma team*, which is now commonplace (although not ubiquitous) in UK hospitals.

Education is central to the recognition and early management of these high risk patients. This should start in medical school with inclusion of intensive care in the core curriculum.[7] It must continue with junior medical and nursing staff by exposure to audit of critical care management. Value should be placed on clinical training within a high dependency unit – these units have been shown to reduce the cardiac arrests in hospital and improve outcome of intensive care units.[8] Fundamental to a more active approach to preventing cardiac arrest will be an ensured availability of high dependency and intensive care resources. It is unacceptable to resuscitate to bed availability.

[5] McQuillan P, Pilkington S, Allan A, *et al.* Confidential inquiry into quality of care before admission to intensive care. *BMJ* 1998;**316**:1853–8.
[6] Nicholl J, Turner J, Dixon S. *The cost-effectiveness of the regional trauma system in the North West Midlands.* Sheffield: Medical Care Unit, University of Sheffield, 1995.
[7] Garrard C, Young D. Suboptimal care of patients before admission to intensive care. *BMJ* 1998;**316**:1841–2.
[8] Franklin C, Rackow E, Mamdami B, *et al.* Decreases in mortality on a large urban medical service by facilitating access to critical care. An alternative to rationing. *Arch Intern Med* 1988;**148**:1403–5.

It is hoped that the rules in this book will help the clinician presented with a critically ill patient to prevent cardiac arrest. Should an arrest occur the clinician might recall important practice points and pitfalls, which will hopefully result in an improved outcome for the patient.

Tim Hodgetts
Nick Castle

Basic
life support

Confidence does not imply competence

The reason

It has been a presumption that professionals who are regularly exposed to resuscitation are competent resuscitators. This presumption may reasonably extend to include doctors (physicians and anaesthetists in particular), nurses, and paramedics. Experience without feedback will increase the confidence to resuscitate, but not the ability.[1]

The confidence of pre-registration house officers in performing resuscitation is artificially inflated by attending cardiac arrests.[1] Competency is confirmed in the mind of the junior doctor after a successful resuscitation, but is rarely questioned when the attempt fails. Medical registrars would be expected to be one of the most skilled groups of doctors in cardiac resuscitation. This group has been shown to be lacking in basic life support skills, knowledge of advanced life support protocols, and the ability to use a defibrillator.[2] Trainee anaesthetists have demonstrated a similar pattern of incompetence.[3] A study of trained nurses failed to identify any nurse who could perform basic life support adequately.[4]

Paediatricians will continue to underperform in the event of cardiac arrest in children if their training is not improved.[5] In a telephone questionnaire survey of middle grade paediatricians, a correct management sequence was offered by only 27% for asystole and only 32% for ventricular fibrillation. A very poor specific knowledge base was identified. In a similar telephone survey of 113 doctors (43 house officers, 50 senior house officers, and 20 registrars) who were members of an adult cardiac arrest team, less than one third could recall the full sequence of management of ventricular fibrillation.[6]

[1] Marteau T, Wynne G, Kaye W, Evans T. Resuscitation: experience without feedback increases confidence but not skill. *BMJ* 1990;**300**:849–50.
[2] David J, Prior-Willeard P. Resuscitation skills of MRCP candidates. *BMJ* 1993;**306**:1578–9.
[3] Bell J, Harrison D, Carr B. Resuscitation skills of trainee anaesthetists. *Anaesth* 1995;**50**:692–4.
[4] Wynne G, Marteau T, Johnston M, Whiteley C, Evans T. Inability of trained nurses to perform basic life support. *BMJ* 1987;**294**:1198–9.
[5] Buss P, Evans R, McCarthy G, Scorrer T, Kumar V. Paediatricians' knowledge of cardiac arrest guidelines. *Arch Dis Child* 1996;**74**:47–9.
[6] Tham K, Evans R, Rubython E, Kinnaird T. Management of ventricular fibrillation by doctors in cardiac arrest teams. *BMJ* 1994;**309**:1408–9.

Learning to resuscitate must be a combination of education and experience, ideally in that order. Feedback to all levels of professional will improve performance.

The exceptions

The development and increasing availability of the *Advanced Life Support* programme (Resuscitation Council UK) has established a standard of practice for hospital-based cardiac resuscitation.[7] The *Advanced Paediatric Life Support*[8] and *Paediatric Advanced Life Support*[9] courses provide training for the less common situation of cardiac arrest in children. A successful candidate must demonstrate a level of knowledge and practical competence in order to pass each of these courses. Confidence is also invariably increased.

However, there will be a predictable degradation of skills after single exposure training, with skills being poorly performed as early as one month following training.[10] Re-accreditation is an essential part of the training and skills retention process. In a study of 280 people aged 11–72 years who had learned cardiopulmonary resuscitation (CPR) from the BBC's 999 training roadshow, an unforewarned video assessment at 6 months in the person's home showed that only 7% could provide safe CPR.[11] Similar results were obtained when 113 medical students were assessed 6 months after a 2-hour CPR training session. There was only a 5% chance that any student would achieve the same mouth-to-mouth ventilation performance.[12] The use of a detailed checklist has been shown to statistically improve the post-course performance of CPR.[10]

[7] Advanced Life Support Course Sub-Committee. Advanced Life Support Course Provider Manual, 3rd edn. London: Resuscitation Council (UK), 1998.

[8] Advanced Life Support Group. *Advanced Paediatric Life Support*, 2nd edn. London: BMJ Publishing, 1997.

[9] Chameides L, Hazinski M (eds). *Pediatric Advanced Life Support*. Dallas: American Heart Association, 1997.

[10] Ward P, Johnson L, Mulligan N, Ward M, Jones D. Improving cardiopulmonary resuscitation skills retention: effect of two checklists designed to prompt correct performance. *Resuscitation* 1997;34:221–5.

[11] Morgan C, Donnelly P, Lester C, Assar D. Effectiveness of the BBC's 999 training roadshow on cardiopulmonary resuscitation. *BMJ* 1996;313:912–6.

[12] Wenzel V, Lehmkuhl P, Kubilis P, *et al*. Poor correlation of mouth-to-mouth ventilation skills after basic life support training and six months later. *Resuscitation* 1997;35:129–34.

You can't start a blue heart*

The reason

Successful resuscitation from a cardiac arrest is dependent upon early recognition of the problem, early access to the emergency services, early basic life support, early defibrillation, and early advanced life support. This is the *Chain of survival*. Firm evidence exists for improved survival with early bystander cardiopulmonary resuscitation (CPR),[1] and early defibrillation.[2,3] The longer the period of hypoxia, the worse the prognosis – with virtually no survival if basic life support is delayed for more than 10 minutes.[4] In a retrospective survey of 414 pre-hospital cardiac arrest patients where no bystander CPR was performed, and it was more than 15 minutes from time of arrest to arrival of an ambulance, there were no survivors to discharge from hospital in the 240 patients with a "non-shockable" rhythm, and one survivor in the "shockable" rhythm group.[5]

Closed chest compressions can only produce blood flows up to 30% of normal cardiac output,[6] but if even a short period of no-flow precedes the initiation of chest compressions the blood flow is borderline for maintaining cerebral viability and restoring heartbeat.[7] Basic life support using closed chest compressions should be regarded as a temporising measure. With few exceptions it will not result in the patient's recovery – although one exception is the apnoea seen after closed head injury without space-occupying haematoma or

* This rule is believed to be first attributed to Dr Douglas Chamberlain, Cardiologist, Brighton, UK.

[1] Scottish Health Service Advisory Council. *Report of the Working Group on Cardiopulmonary Resuscitation (CPR)*. Edinburgh: HMSO, 1993.

[2] Weaver W, Copass M, Bufi D, *et al*. Improved neurolgic recovery and survival after early defibrillation. *Circulation* 1984;**69**:943–8.

[3] Eisenberg M, Copass M, Hallstrom A, *et al*. Treatment of out-of-hospital cardiac arrests with rapid defibrillation by emergency medical technicians. *N Engl J Med* 1980; **302**:1379–83.

[4] Herlitz J, Ekström L, Wennerblom B, *et al*. Effect of bystander initiated cardio-pulmonary resuscitation on ventricular fibrillation and survival after witnessed cardiac arrest outside hospital. *Br Heart J* 1994;**72**:408–12.

[5] Marsden A, Ng G, Dalziel K, Cobbe S. When is it futile for ambulance personnel to initiate cardiopulmonary resuscitation? *BMJ* 1995;**311**:49–51.

[6] Brown C, Werman H. Adrenergic agonists during cardiopulmonary resuscitation. *Resuscitation* 1990;**19**:1–16.

[7] Del Guercio L, Feins N, Cohn J, *et al*. A comparison of blood flow during external and internal cardiac massage in man. *Circulation* 1965;**31**:1171–80.

gross parenchymal disruption, which responds to a few minutes of supportive ventilation.[8] Direct massage of the ventricles by open-chest CPR produces improved coronary and cerebral blood flows. This is because the high right atrial pressure peaks recorded with sternal compressions do not occur with isolated compression of the ventricles.[9] Animal studies have confirmed enhanced coronary blood flow, return of spontaneous circulation, and 24-hour outcome from basic life support with the open compared to the closed technique.[10] Although open-chest CPR has been introduced into the pre-hospital medical system in Belgium, and there was an improvement in return of spontaneous circulation, this was only in cases where closed-chest CPR had failed. There was no long-term conscious survival. In an attempt to make direct heart massage more acceptable to emergency and general physicians a minimally invasive method has been devised, using a pocket-sized plunger-like device introduced through a small intercostal incision.[10,11] This will be one area for future "ultra-advanced life support" research.

It is recognised that, in children, cardiac arrest often involves a period of prolonged hypoxia from respiratory illness before a secondary cardiac arrest. This is reflected in the poor outcome, even when basic life support is started promptly. Early intubation and ventilation with high concentration oxygen is mandatory in the management of these cases.[12]

The exceptions

Congenital heart disease is a rare cause of paediatric cardiac arrest. If resuscitation is successful this will often be despite a right to left shunt and a circulation of predominantly deoxygenated "blue" blood.

[8] Atkinson J, Anderson R, Murray M. The early critical phase of severe head injury: importance of apnea and dysfunctional respiration. *J Trauma* 1998;**45**:941–5.

[9] Tisherman S, Vandevelde K, Safar P, *et al.* Future directions for resuscitation research v ultra-advanced life support. *Resuscitation* 1997;**34**:281–93.

[10] Bircher N, Safar P, Stewart R. A comparison of standard 'MAST'-augmented and open-chest CPR in dogs. A preliminary investigation. *Crit Care Med* 1980;**8**:147–52.

[11] Buckman R, Badellino M, Mauro L, *et al.* Direct cardiac massage without major thoracotomy: feasibility and systemic blood flow. *Resuscitation* 1995;**29**:237–48.

[12] Advanced Life Support Group. Advanced Paediatric Life Support: the practical approach, 2nd edn. London: BMJ Publishing Group, 1996.

If the face is blue, the heart is too

The reason

Cyanosis is a sign of hypoxaemia. During basic life support it may persist for the following reasons:

- Airway obstruction – inability to ventilate beyond a foreign body, laryngeal oedema (burns; direct trauma; anaphylaxis), or an enlarged epiglottis (acute epiglottitis)
- Incorrect airway positioning – inadequate head tilt and chin lift, or inadequate jaw thrust (adults and children >1 year); excessive head tilt, or compression of soft tissues under the jaw during chin lift (infants)
- Insufficient tidal volume – more likely with bag-valve-mask in inexperienced hands, than with mouth-to-mouth or mouth-to-mask (see Rule 6)
- Inadequate chest compressions – too slow, inadequate depth, or incorrect hand positioning.

The exceptions

Central cyanosis is generally only apparent when there is >5 g/100 ml of haemoglobin in the reduced state.[1] If the patient is anaemic, cyanosis may not be seen despite severe hypoxia. Comroe and Botelho pointed out the unreliability of this sign as early as 1947.[2]

An appearance confused with central cyanosis is seen with traumatic asphyxia following hanging, or crushing chest injury. This was first described by Ollivier d'Angers in 1837 as a *masque ecchymotique*. Areas of the body above the level of the heart **and** above the level of compression (head and face following hanging; head, face, neck, upper chest, and upper limbs following chest crush) exhibit widespread petechial haemorrhage. This will persist despite adequate ventilation during resuscitation.

[1] Brewis R. Lecture notes on respiratory disease, 4th edn. Oxford: Blackwell Scientific Publications, 1991.
[2] Comroe J, Botelho S. The unreliability of cyanosis in the recognition of arterial anoxemia. *Am J Med Sci* 1947;**214**:1.

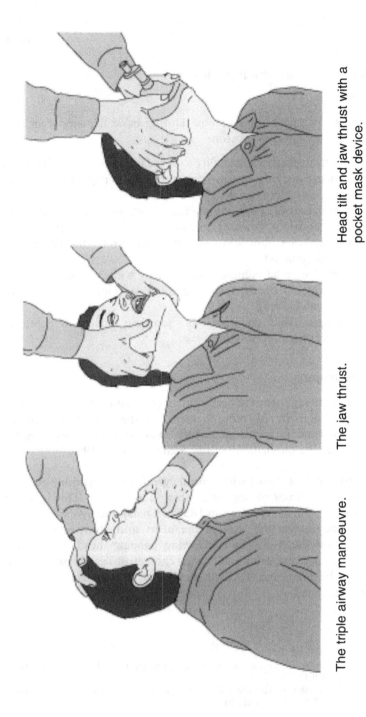

The triple airway manoeuvre.

The jaw thrust.

Head tilt and jaw thrust with a pocket mask device.

An airway is what you do to the head, not what you put in the mouth

The reason

It is a common belief that placing a piece of curved plastic in the mouth (an oropharyngeal or "Guedel" airway) is sufficient to maintain the airway. It is not.

Effective simple airway management involves removing debris by finger sweep or suction, followed by positioning of the head.

The combination of head tilt, chin lift, and mouth open (the *triple airway manoeuvre*) is the most commonly used airway procedure in basic life support. The action of head tilt and chin lift will draw the tongue away from the posterior pharyngeal wall in most cases.

The combination of head tilt, jaw thrust, and mouth open is a more effective way of opening the airway,[1] but it is not conducive to mouth-to-mouth ventilation. It is achievable, however, when performing ventilation using a pocket mask or a bag-valve-mask device.

If trauma to the cervical spine is suspected, the combination of jaw thrust and mouth open is recommended, **without** tilting the head.

The exceptions

When a cuffed airway adjunct is inserted (endotracheal tube, laryngeal mask airway, Combitube) it is not necessary to maintain jaw thrust or head tilt. Indeed, movement of the head following insertion may result in displacement of the tube.

[1] Illingworth K, Simpson K. *Anaesthesia and analgesia in emergency medicine.* Oxford: Oxford University Press, 1994.

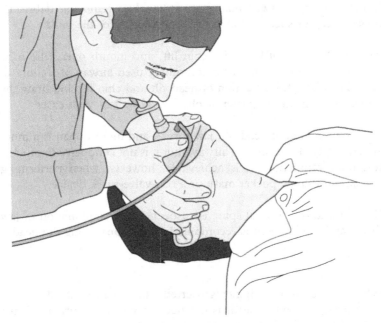

Pocket mask ventilation.

It is better to deliver 17% oxygen to the lungs, than 100% to the back of the throat

The reason

When presented with a choice of using a pocket mask or a bag-valve-mask device to ventilate a patient, there will be a temptation to choose the most sophisticated device in the belief that this will allow improved oxygenation. While a bag-valve-mask with supplementary oxygen and an attached reservoir bag may deliver near 100% oxygen to the lungs in experienced hands, it is a difficult technique for the unpractised (see Rule 8). If the airway is not adequately maintained or there is a poor seal of the mask on the face there may be little, if any, effective ventilation. In this instance it is important to recognise that expired air ventilation (with an oxygen content of ~ 17%) via a pocket mask will sustain the patient. Both hands of the rescuer are used to maintain the seal of the mask, and the capacity of both the rescuer's lungs is available to ensure an adequate tidal volume. The mask of the bag-valve-mask device can be used for this purpose. A *Laerdal Pocket Mask*™ is a superior device that provides a one-way ventilation valve, and optional oxygen port.

The exceptions

Adequate ventilation may be provided by relatively inexperienced staff using a bag-valve-mask when one operator uses both hands to provide a jaw thrust and mask seal, and the other operator squeezes the bag (see Rule 8).

Suction is not catheterisation by the oral route

The reason

Oral suction is an effective way of removing vomit and blood from the upper airway.

There is a tendency to blindly introduce the suction catheter into the mouth (likened to the insertion of a urinary catheter), increasing the risk of laryngeal spasm, vomiting, and in neonates the risk of profound bradycardia.[1]

Suction should be performed with the tip of the suction catheter remaining in direct vision. The tip of a laryngoscope blade may be used to facilitate suction beyond the point of unassisted direct vision.

The exceptions

Tracheal suction via an endotracheal tube or tracheostomy tube *is* performed blind.

[1] Chameides L, Hazinski M (eds). *Pediatric Advanced Life Support.* Dallas: American Heart Association, 1997.

Gasping is not breathing

The reason

It is important not only to recognise a complete absence of respiration, but also to recognise ineffective ventilation. If the respiratory rate is less than 8 breaths/minute in an adult, or if the chest fails to rise on inspiration, then ventilation is ineffective. It is an observation of the authors that CPR has not been started by laypersons (or by trained personnel) because gasping is interpreted as breathing.

Inadequate breathing should be supported by mouth-to-mouth, mouth-to-mask, or bag-valve-mask (see Rule 8) ventilation. In a study of 34 anaesthetised and paralysed patients immediately prior to elective surgery, a tidal volume of 400–600 ml has been shown to be adequate to make the chest rise.[1] This is contrary to earlier recommendations of 800–1200 ml, from the American Heart Association in 1992.[2]

Lower tidal volumes should reduce the risk of gastric insufflation and permit more chest compressions within 1 minute (the target is a rate of 100/minute) because the ventilation fraction of the CPR sequence is shorter.

Importantly, resuscitation training mannequins that are calibrated to the optimal tidal volume of 800–1200 ml should be readjusted.

The exceptions

There are none.

---

[1] Baskett P, Nolan J, Parr M. Tidal volumes which are perceived to be adequate for resuscitation. *Resuscitation* 1996;**31**:231–4.

[2] American Heart Association. Emergency Cardiac Care Committee and Sub-committees. Guidelines for cardiopulmonary resuscitation and emergency cardiac care. Recommendations of the 1992 National Conference. *JAMA* 1992;**268**:2171, 2302.

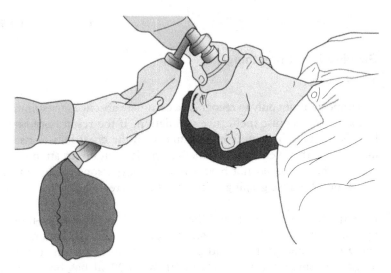

Single operator bag-valve-mask technique.

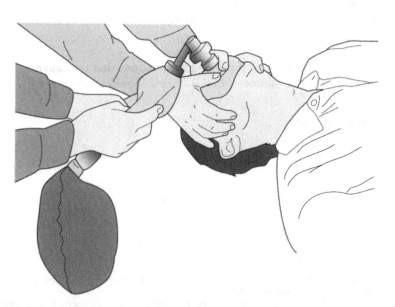

Two-operator bag-valve-mask technique.

Two hands are better than one

The reason

Bag-valve-mask ventilation is a difficult procedure for the in-experienced single operator, and is often performed inadequately.[1] There is commonly a poor seal of the mask with the face[2,3] and poor maintenance of the airway, leading to hypoventilation. This is not improved by aggressive compression of the self-inflating bag, which will only increase gastric insufflation and potential regurgitation.

A two-operator bag-valve-mask technique is recommended.[4] The first operator maintains a jaw thrust and head tilt with two hands, while firmly sealing the mask to the face with both thumbs and index fingers. The second operator provides the ventilation. For optimal oxygenation a reservoir must be used, with a flow rate enough to keep the bag inflated during each ventilation.

A comparison has been made of the tidal volume and mean mask pressures achieved with a single operator or two operators. For the single operator two techniques were used: conventional compression of the bag with one hand; and compression of the bag between the open palm and the side of the body. There was no difference between the single operator techniques, but there was a significantly increased tidal volume and peak mask pressure with the two-person technique.[5]

The exceptions

It is expected that an experienced anaesthetist will have mastery of a one-handed technique – but in an objective assessment of the performance of ambulance officers compared to anaesthetists there was little difference in airway maintenance or mask holding ability in

[1] Seidelin P, Sholarek I, Littelwood D. Comparison of 6 methods of emergency ventilation. *Lancet* 1986;1:1274–5.
[2] Stewart R, Kaplan R, Pennock B, Thompson F. Influence of mask design on bag-mask-ventilation. *Ann Emerg Med* 1985;14:403–6.
[3] Hess D, Baran C. Ventilatory volumes using mouth-to-mouth, mouth-to-mask, and bag-valve-mask techniques. *Respir Care* 1986;31:774–9.
[4] Advanced Life Support Course Sub-Committee. *Advanced Life Support Course Provider Manual*, 3rd edn. London: Resuscitation Council (UK), 1998.
[5] Wheatley S, Thomas A, Taylor R, Brown T. A comparison of three methods of bag valve mask ventilation. *Resuscitation* 1997;33:207–10.

healthy relaxed patients.[6] Importantly, this study was performed on human subjects. Previous studies evaluating the adequacy of pulmonary ventilation during CPR have been on mannequins or lung models.[1,7]

[6] Devitt J, Oakley P, Webster P. Mask lung ventilation by ambulance personnel: a performance assessment. *Can J Anaesth* 1994;41:111–5.
[7] Johannigman J, Branson R, Davis K Jr, Hurst J. Techniques of emergency ventilation: a model to evaluate tidal volume, airway pressure, and gastric insufflation. *J Trauma* 1991;31:93–8.

Only a fool breaks the BLS rule

The reason

Basic life support (BLS) is a drill. It is a sequence of actions that can be performed without question, and with minimum thought. Should the rescuer stop to think, critical steps in the sequence may be omitted.

There are frequently asked questions[1] that must be answered in training to avoid the temptation to stop and think, for example:

- "When do I perform a pre-cordial thump?"
- "Why not do a minute of CPR before going for help?"
- "When should I stop?"

A pre-cordial thump delivers a small amount of energy across the heart that may be adequate to convert ventricular tachycardia (VT) or ventricular fibrillation (VF) into sinus rhythm. It is generally reserved for witnessed and monitored cardiac arrest, in order that those in an organised (yet pulseless) rhythm are not converted into VF or asystole. However, it is possible to imagine a situation where a pre-cordial thump is the *only* treatment that may alter outcome – for example, the hill-walker who suffers an ischaemic cardiac arrest, but is too far from advanced life support (specifically a defibrillator) for it to be effective. In this case it is appropriate to deliver a pre-cordial thump without knowing the rhythm.

It has been estimated that up to 70% of ischaemic cardiac arrests occur in the home. As outcome is inversely related to the time taken to deliver the first defibrillatory shock, it is essential to mobilise the emergency services as rapidly as possible, even at the expense of starting basic life support. The delay in telephoning for an ambulance from the home will be small. The decision whether or not one should abandon the hill-walker to summon help is a dichotomy. The patient will not recover with basic life support alone (see Rule 2), but will equally be irretrievable if one leaves to summon a defibrillator. The reality is that the patient will die whatever action is taken.

[1] Resuscitation Council (UK). *Frequently asked questions on the 1997 resuscitation guidelines for use in the UK*. London: Resuscitation Council (UK), 1997.

The decision whether to start basic life support can be difficult, but the decision to stop can be even more difficult. Reasons to stop are:

- Return of adequate ventilation (see Rule 7) and a palpable central pulse
- Handover to the next echelon of care
- Exhaustion of the rescuer(s).

Prolonged resuscitation attempts may be appropriate in victims of hypothermia, and poisoning (see Rule 26).

The exceptions

The exceptions to starting basic life support are:

- Unsafe environment for the rescuer(s)
- Clearly unsurvivable injuries (for example, decapitation)
- Evidence of extended period since death (rigor mortis, lividity)
- The known existence of an advance directive.

A decision not to start CPR based solely on the patient's age or social status is ethically unacceptable (see Rule 27).

Advanced cardiac life support

Bring the equipment to the patient, not the patient to the equipment

The reason

Medical emergencies can occur anywhere. In hospital, resuscitation equipment is often mobile, for example on trolleys, wall-mounted boxes, or in a rucksack, and can be brought to the patient's bedside on the ward or to where the patient is found collapsed in the corridor, toilet, or car park. Flexibility in response can be lost when resuscitation equipment is stationary – for example, when fixed to the wall of the resuscitation room in the accident and emergency department.

The critical aspects in cardiac arrest outcome are the provision of early basic life support[1-3] and early defibrillation.[4-6] Should a patient suffer a cardiac arrest outside a clinical area, CPR should be started and the defibrillator brought to the patient. If the patient is placed on a trolley and rushed to the equipment, there are two principal problems:

1 There will be no effective basic life support during the transfer.
2 Poor airway control during the transfer may result in avoidable aspiration.

The exceptions

Sometimes it is not appropriate to bring the equipment to the patient. These are invariably situations where the safety of the rescuer is threatened, and the patient must first be moved to a place of safety (the near-drowning casualty who is still in the water; the injured patient who has fallen downstairs disorientated by the smoke in a burning building).

[1] Eisenberg M, Bergner L, Hallstrom A. Cardiac resuscitation in the community. *JAMA* 1979;**241**:1905–7.
[2] Thompson R, Hallstrom A, Cobb L. Bystander-initiated cardiopulmonary resuscitation in the management of ventricular fibrillation. *Ann Intern Med* 1979;**90**:737–40.
[3] Copley D, Mantle J, Rogers W, *et al.* Improved outcome for prehospital cardio-pulmonary collapse with resuscitation by bystanders. *Circulation* 1977;**56**:901–5.
[4] Stults K, Brown D, Schug V, Bean J. Prehospital defibrillation performed by emergency medical technicians in rural communities. *N Engl J Med* 1984;**310**:219–23.
[5] Cobbe S, Redmond M, Watson J, Hollingworth J, Carrington D. "Heartstart Scotland" – initial experience of a national scheme for out of hospital defibrillation. *BMJ* 1991; **302**:1517–20.
[6] Pionkowski R, Thompson B, Gruchow H, Aprahamian C, Darin J. Resuscitation time in ventricular fibrillation – a prognostic indicator. *Ann Emerg Med* 1983;**12**:733–8.

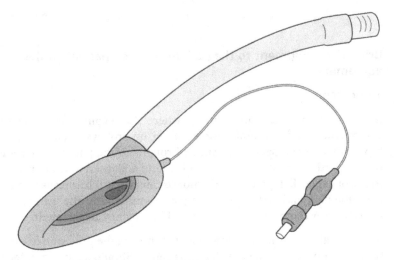

A laryngeal mask airway (LMA).

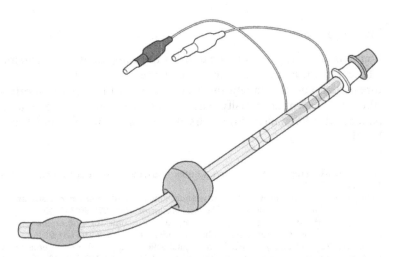

A Combitube.

The laryngoscope is an oxygen deprivation device

The reason

As long as the laryngoscope is in the patient's mouth, the patient is not receiving oxygen.

It is recommended that each intubation attempt should take no longer than 30 seconds. The patient must be reoxygenated by bag-valve-mask technique between attempts. Take a deep breath in, breathe out and hold your breath (your patient is holding their breath in expiration) as the laryngoscope is picked up – if you need to breathe, then so does the patient.

The problem is compounded in children, who have a higher respiratory rate and less functional residual capacity than adults. Children cannot hold their breath for as long as adults, and will tolerate this iatrogenic hypoventilation less well.

The exceptions

Endotracheal intubation remains the standard for definitive airway management. Laryngoscopy is necessary to achieve this. Alternatives to endotracheal intubation are available (see Rule 12), which do not require laryngoscopy and include:

- Laryngeal mask airway (LMA)
- Combitube.

Both of these alternatives allow assisted ventilation via a bag-valve device. Neither is as completely reliable as the endotracheal tube in preventing inhalation of gastric contents.

Rule 12

Save the day with an LMA

The reason

Effective ventilation and oxygenation is essential for a successful outcome from cardiac arrest, but to achieve this while maintaining the airway by manual techniques is difficult (see Rule 4 and Rule 8). Endotracheal intubation is regarded as the "gold standard" technique to secure the airway, but it is a complex skill to learn and requires regular practice. The common result at a cardiac arrest is that simple techniques are variably applied to maintain an unprotected airway.

Insertion of a laryngeal mask airway (LMA) is a simpler skill to learn than endotracheal intubation.[1] It has reportedly been taught to paramedics in as little as 1 minute,[2] but the recommendations from the Joint Colleges Ambulance Liaison Committee are for 2–3 hours theoretical and mannequin training, followed by 5 successful insertions in a live patient.[3] The LMA is available in adult and paediatric sizes and is reusable, unlike the Combitube (see below). Reports of aspiration of gastric contents are few[4] and in one prospective study of 2359 cases there were two patients who regurgitated, but without any sequelae from aspiration.[5] Recurrent laryngeal nerve palsy is a reported complication.[6]

There are attractions for the LMA in pre-hospital care because of the reduced practice for endotracheal intubation (it has replaced the endotracheal tube in over 50% of surgical procedures[1]), and the reduced need to tilt the head when inserted in a patient with potential cervical spine injury (a cervical collar or manual immobilisation have been shown not to interfere with insertion[7]).

[1] Sasada M, Gabbott D. The role of the laryngeal mask airway in pre-hospital care. *Resuscitation* 1994;**28**:97–102.

[2] Pennant J, Walker M. Comparison of the endotracheal tube and laryngeal mask in airway management by paramedical personnel. *Anesth Analg* 1992;**74**:531–4.

[3] Joint Colleges Ambulance Liaison Committee. The use of the laryngeal mask airway. *Today's Emergency* 1998;**4**:39.

[4] Griffin R, Hatcher I. Aspiration pneumonia and the laryngeal mask airway. *Anaesth* 1990;**45**:1039–40.

[5] Verghese C, Smith T, Young E. Prospective survey of the use of the laryngeal mask airway in 2359 patients. *Anaesth* 1993;**48**:58–60

[6] Lloyd Jones F, Hegab A. Recurrent laryngeal nerve palsy after laryngeal mask airway insertion. *Anaesth* 1996;**51**:171–2.

[7] Pennant J, Pace N, Gajraj N. Role of the laryngeal mask airway in the immobile cervical spine. *J Clin Anesth* 1993;**5**:226–30.

In a multi-centre hospital trial to assess the value of the LMA when used by ward nurses during the early phase of resuscitation, nurses were given 90 minutes of theory training and were then supervised to achieve five successful LMA insertions in the operating theatre. At subsequent cardiac arrests on the ward the LMA was inserted at the first attempt in 71% of cases, and at the second attempt in 26%. The mean interval from cardiac arrest to LMA insertion was 2·4 minutes. Regurgitation occurred *before* the LMA was inserted in 12% (20 cases), and *during* the insertion in 2% (3 cases), but there was clinical evidence of aspiration in only 1 case.[8]

The exceptions

A further recommended alternative to endotracheal intubation is the Combitube.[9] Like the LMA, this device does not require laryngoscopy for insertion. The device has been evaluated for pre-hospital use by paramedics where it is recommended as a back-up to endotracheal intubation, and as a primary airway. In a prospective field trial of 52 patients in cardiac arrest the Combitube was inserted successfully in 71% of cases when it was used as a primary airway, and in 64% of cases who could not be intubated by the conventional method. However, in a follow-up survey at 15 months, 9 of 11 randomly selected paramedics showed inadequate skill retention.[10]

In a trial of 470 cases of pre-hospital cardiac and/or respiratory arrest the Combitube was compared with the LMA and the pharyngeal tracheal lumen airway (PTLA – similar in concept to the Combitube, but slightly different design). Successful intubation and ventilation was achieved by paramedics in 86% with Combitube, 82% with PTLA, and 73% with LMA. The Combitube was associated with the least problems with ventilation, and was the preferred airway adjunct by the majority of paramedics.[11]

[8] Stone B, Leach A, Alexander C, *et al.* The use of the laryngeal mask airway by nurses during cardiopulmonary resuscitation. *Anaesth* 1994;**49**:3–7.
[9] Advanced Life Support Course Sub-Committee. *Advanced Life Support Course Provider Manual*, 3rd edn. London: Resuscitation Council (UK), 1998.
[10] Atherton G, Johnson J. Ability of paramedics to use the Combitube in pre-hospital cardiac arrest. *Ann Emerg Med* 1993;**22**:1263–8.
[11] Rumball C, MacDonald D. The PTL, laryngeal mask and oral airway: a randomized pre-hospital comparative study of ventilatory device effectiveness and cost-effectiveness in 470 cases of cardiorespiratory arrest. *Prehospital Emerg Care* 1997;**1**:1–10.

Additional success in hospital has been reported where the Combitube has secured the airway when endotracheal intubation has failed in a patient with a bull neck,[12] and failure to visualise the cords because of blood or vomit.[13,14]

Recognised complications of the Combitube are oesophageal perforation[15] and tracheal perforation.

[12] Banyai M, Falger S, Roggla M, *et al*. Emergency intubation with the Combitube in a grossly obese patient with a bull neck. *Resuscitation* 1993;**26**:271–6.

[13] Klauser R, Roggla G, Pidlich J, Leithner C, Frass M. Massive upper airway bleeding after thrombolytic therapy: successful airway management with the Combitube. *Ann Emerg Med* 1992;**21**:431–3.

[14] Staudinger T, Tesinsky P, Klappacher G, *et al*. Emergency intubation with the Combitube in two cases of difficult airway management. *Eur J Anaesth* 1995;**12**:189–93.

[15] Vézina D, Lessard M, Bussières J, Topping C, Trépanier C. Complications associated with the use of the Esophageal-Tracheal Combitube. *Can J Anaesth* 1998;**45**:76–80.

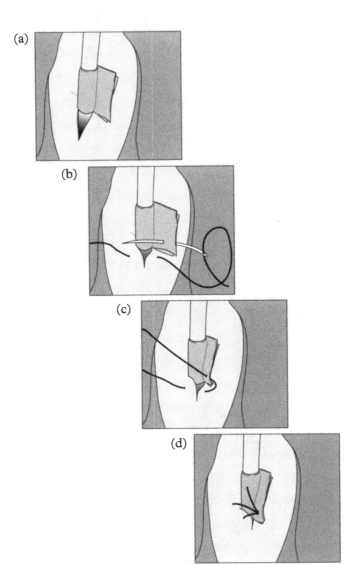

Steps for securing a chest drain with a tape flag.

(a) Pull the chest drain to one end of the wound
(b) Take a 6 cm strip of woven tape (elastoplast or zinc oxide) and fold around the tube flush with the skin, to make a "flag"
(c) Place a suture through the wound and the tape flag
(d) Secure with a knot

If you can put it in, you can pull it out

The reason

The transfer of a patient pre-hospital, intra-hospital, or inter-hospital represents a period of risk. Not only is the patient at risk of deterioration, but there is a significant risk of losing an intravenous line, an endotracheal tube, a chest drain, or an arterial line. To avoid these complications the following steps should be taken:

- Endotracheal tubes should be secured using non-elasticated bandage (elasticated bandage may stretch and become loose)
- Secure all intravenous cannulae* with tape or a proprietary dressing, then loop each giving set and tape to the skin to provide additional security – then bandage over each cannula
- Obtain a second intravenous access line in case the first fails
- Protect an intraosseous line with a box splint (see Rule 55)
- Use a tape flag to rapidly and effectively secure a chest drain
- Tape the drainage tubing of a urinary catheter to the patient's leg, to prevent untoward traction on the catheter balloon
- Ensure any patient who is lifted on a spinal board is adequately secured. The patient is balancing on seven points of contact (occiput, scapulae, ischial tuberosities, heels) on a slippery surface.

The exceptions

Any doubt about the position of an endotracheal tube warrants its immediate removal and a return to bag-valve-mask ventilation – *when in doubt, take it out.*

---

* There is a tendency to tape intravenous lines neatly, but insecurely. Neatness can be addressed once the patient arrives at the definitive care facility.

Oxygen is free – don't make your patient work for it

The reason

Hypoxia is a common finding in patients immediately prior to admission to the intensive care unit.[1] The reasons identified are a failure of system organisation, a lack of clinical knowledge of medical staff, a failure to appreciate clinical urgency (and therefore a late referral to the intensive care unit), a lack of supervision of junior medical staff, and a failure to seek advice.

Oxygen by face-mask is often withheld because of an irrational fear of adversely depressing respiration in the small proportion of chronic bronchitics whose respiration centre is stimulated by hypoxia (so-called "hypoxic drive"). This denies the majority of patients the oxygen they need. Remember, it is not oxygen that kills, but lack of oxygen.

It is a frequently observed practice for a bag-valve-mask system to be used as an oxygen delivery system. This is a secondary purpose for which it was designed, and has important limitations. To establish any oxygen flow the patient must open the demand valve, which requires $\sim 0.75 \, cmH_2O$ inspiratory pressure with an oxygen flow rate of 15 L/min (or $1.5 \, cmH_2O$ at 30 L/min and $3 \, cmH_2O$ at 60 L/min).[2] This may not be achieved in a patient in respiratory distress, particularly one who is tiring. The reason this system is used is in the mistaken belief that it is comparable to a Waters' bag (see Rule 15). A Waters' circuit does not contain a valve between the bag and the mask, thereby reducing the resistance to inspiration, but it does have its own problems in the resuscitation situation.

High flow oxygen by a partial non-rebreathing mask with reservoir should be the standard for oxygen delivery in spontaneously breathing critically ill patients.

[1] McQuillan P, Pilkington S, Allan A, et al. Confidential inquiry into quality of care before admission to intensive care. BMJ 1998;316:1853–8.
[2] Personal communication. The inspiration breathing resistance of a Laerdal patient valve. Smiths Industries Medical Systems, January 1999.

The exceptions

Oxygen can be a scarce resource, for example in a military operational environment. The World Health Organization has recommended the criteria for giving oxygen to children with respiratory infections in the third world to be:[3]

- Cyanosis
- Inability to drink
- Severe intercostal recession
- Respiratory rate of >70 breaths/minute.

These criteria have independently been found to predict hypoxaemia with a sensitivity of 62%.[4] The case fatality rate of pneumonia is directly related to hypoxaemia.[5]

A small proportion of chronic bronchitics are reliant on hypoxic drive – the so-called "blue bloater". These patients should be given 24% oxygen initially, and have further oxygen therapy dictated by blood gas analysis.

[3] WHO Programme for the control of acute respiratory infections. *Oxygen therapy for acute respiratory infections in young children in developing countries.* Geneva: WHO/ARI/ 90.5, 1993.
[4] Weber M, Usen S, Palmer A, Jaffar S, Mulholland E. Predictors of hypoxaemia in hospital admissions with acute lower respiratory tract infection in a developing country. *Arch Dis Child* 1997;76:310–14.
[5] Onyango F, Steinhoff M, Wafula E, Wariua S, Musia J, Kitonyi J. Hypoxaemia in young Kenyan children with acute lower respiratory tract infection. *BMJ* 1993;306: 612–5.

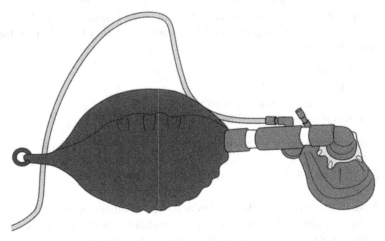

A Waters' bag to deliver "100%" oxygen.

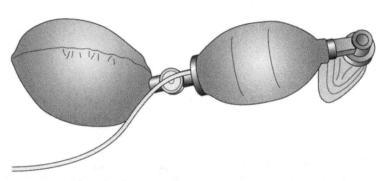

A bag-valve-mask apparatus to deliver "100%" oxygen.

You are in deep Waters when the oxygen runs out

The reason

A Waters' circuit is popular with anaesthetists. It comprises of a collapsible rubber bag that will inflate with oxygen from a cylinder or wall source. The variable resistance in the expiration valve can be used to control inflation pressures on compression of the bag. The device is commonly connected to an advanced airway adjunct (usually an endotracheal tube), rather than to a contoured hard rubber facemask (often only available where there are full anaesthetic facilities). A Waters' bag* offers a superior "feel" over a bag-valve-mask apparatus. As no atmospheric air is entrained it provides 100% oxygen at the alveoli.

There are two principal problems with using a Waters' bag:

1   It is unsuitable for use by the inexperienced single operator, as practice is required to master single-handed airway control while squeezing the bag (see Rule 6).
2   A Waters' bag cannot function without an oxygen supply. It is **not** therefore suitable as the primary equipment for ventilation in emergency situations where the oxygen supply may be interrupted – specifically, where cylindered oxygen is being used (pre-hospital care; mobile resuscitation trolleys on wards; intra-hospital transfer of patients).

The exceptions

Incorrect bag-valve-mask technique is associated with pulmonary barotrauma and the development of simple or tension pneumothorax.[1-3] This is reported when positive pressure is maintained during the relaxation phase of the bag (that is, the grip is incompletely released), or when the reservoir is overfilled or its opening is partially occluded.[3]

---

* After Ralph M Waters (b. 1883), pioneer anaesthetist, University of Wisconsin.

[1] Hillman K, Albin M. Pulmonary barotrauma during cardiopulmonary resuscitation. *Crit Care Med* 1986;14:606.
[2] Tucker J, Hanson C, Chen L. Pneumothorax re-exacerbated by a self-inflating bag-valve device. *Anaesthesiology* 1992;76:1067.
[3] Silbergleit R, Lee D, Blank-Reid C, McNamara R. Sudden severe barotrauma from self-inflating bag-valve devices. *J Trauma* 1996;40:320-2.

Rule 16

Treat the patient, not the monitor

The reason

Any apparent change in cardiac rhythm requires, as a first action, the status of the patient to be checked.

If the default setting of a monitor-defibrillator is "paddles", then apparent *asystole* will be seen (a straight line, unlike the slow undulating line of true physiological asystole) irrespective of the true rhythm when the machine is turned on, unless the paddles are placed on the chest. To avoid misinterpretation many modern monitor-defibrillators will display a broken line and the caption "PADDLES" to warn the operator.

Asystole will also be seen on the monitor if an ECG lead becomes disconnected. This is **electrical asystole** and appears as a completely straight line. **Physiological asystole** has a slowly undulating baseline. If Tutankhamun were to be connected to a monitor, there would be a slowly undulating baseline. When asystole is seen, check the leads and check the patient.

An appearance resembling ventricular fibrillation may be produced on the monitor by vigorously shaking the leads (for example, the patient who is connected to the monitor and brushing his teeth at the sink), or by muscular contractions during an epileptic convulsion or shivering. A failure to check the patient may mean an inappropriate shock at best, or a fatal error at worst.

In a busy resuscitation area with adjacent monitored patients, it is even possible to treat the monitor attached to a different patient.

The exceptions

The 1997 European Resuscitation Council guidelines for advanced cardiac life support do not require a pulse check between direct current shocks for ventricular fibrillation.[1] If there is no change in rhythm a further shock within a three-shock sequence may be given

[1] Kloeck W, Cummins R, Chamberlain D, Bossaert L, Callanan V, *et al.* The universal ALS algorithm. *Resuscitation* 1997;34:109–11.

without the pulse check. In other words, the monitor dictates the action. Pulse checks are not required after the first direct current shock given for pulseless ventricular tachycardia if the waveform remains the same.[2] Pulse checks **are** recommended between subsequent shocks.

[2] Robertson C, Steen P, Adgey J, Bossaert L, Carli P. The 1998 European Resuscitation Council guidelines for adult advanced life support. *Resuscitation* 1998;37:81–90.

Paddles in, people out – paddles out, people in

The reason

Doctors, nurses, and ambulance personnel who are regularly involved with cardiac resuscitation become accustomed to automatically stand back from the patient when the paddles of a manual defibrillator are placed on the patient's chest. Removal of the paddles from the chest is the non-verbal signal for personnel to step towards the patient and continue with basic and advanced life support.

If the rhythm changes to a "non-shockable" rhythm when the defibrillator is being charged with the paddles on the chest, the paddles must be replaced on the defibrillator and the charge dumped (for example, by turning the monitor-defibrillator off, or by changing the selected energy setting). This means that live paddles will be moved away from the patient as the rest of the team moves towards the patient. An authoritative warning must be given – *"Stand clear! Live paddles!"*

The exceptions

Automatic external defibrillators, or AEDs (see Rule 19), utilise large adhesive electrodes which record the rhythm (the computer then analyses the rhythm, in a consistently more sensitive manner than the naked eye) and deliver direct current shocks when appropriate. The machines often provide a warning voice message to "Stand clear" before defibrillation. These hands-free defibrillators are intrinsically safer for the operator to use than the manual defibrillator.

However, an inappropriate shock may be administered to the patient when there is considerable electrical interference that is interpreted as ventricular fibrillation, for example during an epileptic convulsion. Manual override keys are available, and when used may provide another opportunity for the defibrillator to be charged inappropriately.

Pray when you defibrillate

The reason

Firm pressure through the electrode paddles during defibrillation contributes to reducing the transthoracic impedance (resistance of the chest wall) and increases the probability of successful cardioversion.[1-3] If you hold your hands together as if praying and press as hard as you can, this is the pressure you should generate on the chest wall (which approximates to the recommended 10 kg[4])!

Additional factors that contribute to reducing the transthoracic impedance are:

* A salt-containing coupling agent (defibrillation gel pads)
* Shock delivery during end expiration
* Large electrode paddle size
* A short time interval between successive shocks.

It is important that the rescuer managing the airway resists the temptation to provide a ventilation immediately prior to defibrillation, as this will increase the chest wall resistance. In paediatric resuscitation the adult electrodes (13 cm diameter) should be used as soon as the chest size permits, which will be approximately at 10 kg or one year old.[5,6]

If the polarity of the current is reversed part way through the delivery of the shock, a smaller energy is required for successful defibrillation. This is the principle of the *biphasic defibrillator,* which is the technology behind automatic implantable defibrillators. The potential for smaller,

[1] Kerber R, Jensen S, Grayzel J, Hoyt R, Kennedy J. Determinants of defibrillation: prospective analysis of 183 patients. *Am J Cardiol* 1983;**52**:739–45.
[2] Kerber R, Grayzel J, Hoyt R, Marcus M, Kennedy J. Transthoracic resistance in human defibrillation. Influence of body weight, chest size, serial shocks, paddle size and paddle contact pressure. *Circulation* 1981;**63**:676–82.
[3] Sirna S, Ferguson D, Charbonnier F, Kerber R. Factors affecting transthoracic impedance during electrical cardioversion. *Am J Cardiol* 1988;**62**:1048–52.
[4] Advanced Life Support Course Sub-Committee. *Advanced Life Support Course Provider Manual,* 3rd edn. London: Resuscitation Council (UK), 1998.
[5] Atkins D, Sirna S, Kieso R, Charbonnier F, Kerber R. Pediatric defibrillation: importance of paddle size in determining transthoracic impedance. *Pediatr* 1988;**82**:914–8.
[6] Atkins D, Kerber R. Pediatric defibrillation: current flow is improved by using "adult" electrode paddles. *Pediatr* 1994;**94**:90–3.

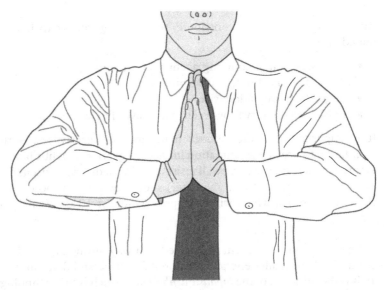

Pray when you defibrillate.

safer automatic external and manual defibrillators is currently under development.

The exceptions

The automatic external defibrillator (AED) is a "hands free" device. The emphasis of the AED is simplicity and rescuer safety. There is no opportunity to apply pressure through the adhesive electrodes.

An AED in your hands is worth two manuals in a rush

The reason

The automatic external defibrillator (AED) was first described in 1979.[1] AEDs accurately detect ventricular fibrillation (VF) and ventricular tachycardia (VT) in adults[2] and children over 8 years old.[3] They can be used successfully by minimally trained personnel.[2,4]

The value of early defibrillation by ambulance personnel is well recorded (see Rule 2). A substantial increase in survival is documented when AEDs are used in an urban setting compared to a manual defibrillator.[5] This has been attributed to a reduced time to shock delivery.[6]

AEDs are now so portable, simple to use, and rapid to respond that they are part of the American Heart Association's Basic Cardiac Life Support course, and are not restricted to health care professionals. They have become increasingly available to basic trained non-medical staff including voluntary aid society personnel,[7] the military,[8] supermarket employees, and aircraft attendants. Placement of an AED in the home of a high risk patient (a survivor of cardiac arrest) for use by a relative has also been advocated.[9,10]

[1] Diack A, Welborn W, Rullman R, Walter C, Wayne M. An automatic cardiac resuscitator for emergency treatment of cardiac arrest. *Med Instrum* 1979;**13**:78–83.

[2] Cummins R, Eisenberg M, Bergner L, Murray J. Sensitivity, accuracy and safety of an automatic external defibrillator. *Lancet* 1984;**2**:318–20.

[3] Atkins D, Hartley L, York D. Accurate recognition and effective treatment of ventricular fibrillation by automated external defibrillators in adolescents. *Pediatr* 1998; **101**:393–7.

[4] Stukts K, Brown D, Kerber R. Efficacy of an automated external defibrillator in the management of out-of-hospital cardiac arrest: validation of the diagnostic algorithm and initial clinical experience in a rural environment. *Circulation* 1986;**73**:701–9.

[5] Weaver W, Hill D, Fahrenbruch C, *et al.* Use of the automatic external defibrillator in the management of out-of-hospital cardiac arrest. *N Engl J Med* 1988;**319**:661–6.

[6] Cummins R, Eisenberg M, Litwin P, Graves J, Hearne T, Hallstrom A. Automatic external defibrillators used by emergency medical technicians: a controlled clinical trial. *JAMA* 1987;**257**:1605–10.

[7] Walters G, Glucksman E, Evans T. Training St John Ambulance volunteers to use an automated external defibrillator. *Resuscitation* 1994;**27**:39–45.

[8] Ten Eyck R. Automated external defibrillator training and skills maintenance in Air Force emergency medical service systems. *Milit Med* 1993;**158**:579–81.

[9] Moore J, Eisenberg M, Andresen E, *et al.* Home placement of automatic external defibrillators among survivors of ventricular fibrillation. *Ann Emerg Med* 1986;**15**: 811–2.

[10] Moore J, Eisenberg M, Cummins R, Hallstrom A, Litwin P. Lay person use of automatic external defibrillation. *Ann Emerg Med* 1987;**16**:669–72.

The·particular benefit of utilising the police as first responders with a defibrillation capability has been noted. In a prospective analysis of police and ambulance response times in Minnesota, police arrived at the cardiac arrest 1–2 minutes before the ambulance in 34% of cases.[11] In a follow-up study when police were trained to use an AED there was a high discharge home survival rate (13 of 31 patients had return of spontaneous circulation with police defibrillation, all surviving to discharge, and 5 others survived to discharge after advanced life support from ambulance paramedics).[12]

The exceptions

An AED will detect and deliver sequential shocks to VF and VT (but an AED will not deliver a shock to a broad complex tachycardia with a rate <150 beats per minute). There are circumstances where it is also necessary to cardiovert narrow complex tachydysrhythmias (atrial fibrillation, atrial flutter, supraventricular tachycardia) although it is recognised that this would be appropriate pre-hospital in only extremely limited situations. An AED can be converted to manual mode with an override key. However, wide availability of such keys may encourage subjective opinion to override the sensitive and accurate computer programmes – their use should be confined to appropriately experienced personnel.

A *shock advisory* defibrillator automatically detects VF or VT, but requires the operator to deliver the shock after a verbal computer-generated instruction. The electrode pads are similar to the AED.

[11] White R, Vukov L, Bugliosi T. Early defibrillation by police: initial experience with measurement of critical time intervals and patient outcome. *Ann Emerg Med* 1994;23: 1009–13.
[12] White R, Asplin B, Bugliosi T, Hankins D. High discharge survival rate after out-of-hospital ventricular fibrillation with rapid defibrillation by police and paramedics. *Ann Emerg Med* 1996;28:480–5.

When it's going down the tubes think of your NAVAL

The reason

Intravenous access can sometimes be difficult to achieve in a cardiac arrest or medical emergency. This is predictable when the rescuer is inexperienced in cannulation, or the patient is hypothermic, hypovolaemic, or an intravenous drug abuser. In situations where drugs are needed immediately and the airway is secured by an endotracheal tube, the following may be given down the tube:[1]

- N Naloxone
- A Adrenaline (epinephrine)
- V Valium*
- A Atropine
- L Lignocaine

*This is the proprietary name for diazepam solution – the emulsion (Diazemuls) is unsuitable for the endotracheal route.

In order to obtain similar plasma concentrations to the intravenous route, it is recommended to double or treble the dose.[2] While it is important to have sufficient volume for the drug to be dispersed to the alveoli for absorption, this must be balanced against administering an excessive volume (for example, atropine 6 mg given in asystole should be as 2 × 3 mg in 10 ml doses, not 6 × 1 mg in 10 ml). Theoretically, in a patient lying supine with a curved endotracheal tube *in situ*, drugs given down the tube may accumulate in the "U" bend. To counter this, proprietary tracheal drug introducers are available (long, fine, stiffened catheters with a small distal rose to spray the drug). These have not been shown to be any more effective than simple administration into the endotracheal tube. However, it is recommended to follow any endotracheal drug with 5–10 ventilations to assist dispersal.[3]

[1] Allison E, Hunt R, Gardner M, Prasad N. *Advanced Life Support Skills*. St Louis: Mosby Year Books, 1994.
[2] Advanced Life Support Course Sub-Committee. *Advanced Life Support Course Provider Manual*, 3rd edn. London: Resuscitation Council (UK), 1998.
[3] Robertson C, Steen P, Adgey J, Bossaert L, Carli P. The 1998 European Resuscitation Council guidelines for adult advanced life support. *Resuscitation* 1998;37:81–90.

The exceptions

It is contraindicated to give either sodium bicarbonate or calcium chloride (or calcium gluconate) down the endotracheal tube. In adults, proceed to central venous cannulation to administer these drugs.

When peripheral intravenous access fails in children, think immediately of the intraosseous route (see Rule 55).

There is no drug that will convert VF to sinus rhythm

The reason

Adrenaline (epinephrine) is the principal drug in the current European Resuscitation Council[1] and American Heart Association[2] guidelines for the management of cardiac arrest in adults and children. It was first proposed for use in cardiac arrest in 1896,[3] and has survived repeated revisions of advanced cardiac life support algorithms when other drugs have been relegated in importance (sodium bicarbonate, calcium chloride) or removed altogether (isoprenaline).

However, no drug (including adrenaline (epinephrine)) can convert the commonest primary cardiac arrest dysrhythmia (ventricular fibrillation) to sinus rhythm – nor has any drug been shown to affect the outcome from cardiac arrest. The only proven interventions that reduce mortality in this situation are early basic life support[4] and early defibrillation.[5]

Early small studies to investigate the benefit of high dose adrenaline (epinephrine) (5–10 mg intravenously) were encouraging[6,7] and a pre-hospital prospective randomised controlled trial showed a significant

[1] Advanced Life Support Working Group of the European Resuscitation Council. The 1998 European Resuscitation Council guidelines for adult advanced life support. *BMJ* 1998;**316**:1863–9.

[2] Emergency cardiac care committee and subcommittees, American Heart Association. Guidelines for cardiopulmonary resuscitation and emergency cardiac care. *JAMA* 1992;**268**:2199–241.

[3] Gottlieb R. Ueber die wirkung der nebennierenextract auf herz und blutdruck. *Arch Exp Pathol Pharmakol* 1896;**38**:99–112.

[4] Scottish Health Service Advisory Council. Report of the Working Group on Cardiopulmonary Resuscitation (CPR). Edinburgh: HMSO, 1993.

[5] Weaver W, Copass M, Bufi D, *et al.* Improved neurolgic recovery and survival after early defibrillation. *Circulation* 1984;**69**:943–8.

[6] Barton C, Callaham M. High-dose epinephrine improves the return of spontaneous circulation rates in human victims of cardiac arrest. *Ann Emerg Med* 1991;**20**:722–5.

[7] Lindner K, Ahnfield F, Prengel A. Comparison of standard and high-dose adrenaline in the resuscitation of asystole and electromechanical dissociation. *Acta Anaesthesiol Scand* 1991;**35**:253–6.

improvement in early outcome measures.[8] However, this has not been reproduced in three subsequent large trials,[9-11] and there is no increased survival at 6 months compared to the standard dose adrenaline (epinephrine) group.[11]

The exceptions

Why should so much importance continue to be placed on adrenaline (epinephrine)? In the fibrillating heart, adrenaline (epinephrine) may increase the amplitude and frequency of the fibrillating waveform,[12] and may also reduce the threshold for fibrillation.[13] A theoretical benefit is the preferential distribution of available arterial supply to vital organs, such as the heart and brain.[1] In this context, adrenaline (epinephrine) is an adjunct to basic life support.

Despite these physiological benefits, Rainer *et al.* deduce from a review of the available literature that much of the evidence is inconclusive, but, if anything, adrenaline (epinephrine) is associated with *poorer* outcomes.[14]

[8] Callaham M, Madsen C, Barton C, Saunders C, Pointer J. A randomised clinical trial of high-dose epinephrine and norepinephrine vs standard-dose epinephrine in prehospital cardiac arrest. *JAMA* 1992;**21**:2667–72.

[9] Stiell I, Herbert P, Weitzman B, *et al.* High-dose epinephrine in adult cardiac arrest. *N Engl J Med* 1992;**327**:1045–50.

[10] Brown C, Martin D, Pepe P, *et al.* Multicenter High-dose Epinephrine Study Group. A comparison of standard-dose and high-dose epinephrine in cardiac arrest outside the hospital. *N Engl J Med* 1992;**327**:1051–5.

[11] Choux C, Gueugniaud P-Y, Barbiuex A, *et al.* Standard doses versus repeated high doses of epinephrine in cardiac arrest outside the hospital. *Resuscitation* 1995;**29**:3–9.

[12] Livesay J, Folette D, Fey K, *et al.* Optimising myocardial supply/demand balance with alpha-adrenergic drugs during cardiopulmonary resuscitation. *J Thorac Cardiovasc Surg* 1978;**76**:244–51.

[13] Ruffy R, Schechtman K, Monje E. β-adrenergic modulation of direct fibrillation energy in anaesthetised dog heart. *Am J Physiol* 1985;**248**:H674–7.

[14] Rainer T, Robertson C. Adrenaline, cardiac arrest, and evidence based medicine. *J Accid Emerg Med* 1996;**13**:234–7.

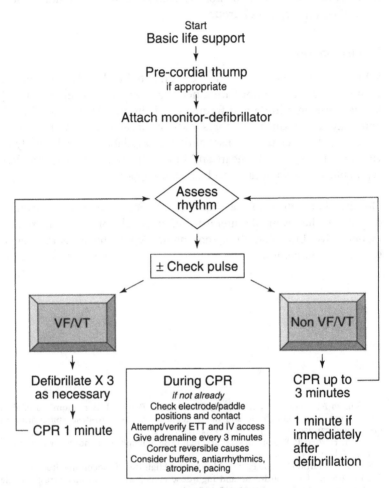

The cardiac arrest rhythm treatment algorithm.

Think of the causes to begin and treat them if you want to win

. . . . . or your patient is for THE CHOP

The reason

There are a number of potentially treatable causes of cardiac arrest when the diagnosis is electromechanical dissociation (EMD) – also known as pulseless electrical activity (PEA).

There are two ways of remembering the causes: choose the one you prefer.

	THE CHOP		4 Hs and 4 Ts
T	Tension pneumothorax	H	Hypoxia
H	Hypovolaemia	H	Hypovolaemia
E	Electrolyte imbalance	H	Hypo-/Hyperkalaemia
		H	Hypothermia
C	Cardiac tamponade	T	Tamponade (cardiac)
H	Hypothermia	T	Tension pneumothorax
O	Overdose	T	Toxic disturbances (overdose)
P	Pulmonary embolus	T	Thromboembolic/mechanical obstruction

It is impractical to look for and treat all potential causes simultaneously. Start the "non-VF/VT" protocol (see diagram),[1] then consider each cause sequentially in the first and subsequent loops.

The exceptions

Organised electrical activity without a pulse is commonly seen following defibrillation, during a continued attempt to resuscitate the patient. It may occur without any of the treatable causes as an agonal (terminal rhythm).

[1] Adapted from: The 1998 European Resuscitation Council guidelines for adult advanced life support. *BMJ* 1998;**316**:1863–9.

Adenosine, shut that door!

The reason

Supraventricular tachycardia (SVT) describes any regular tachycardia arising above the ventricles in excess of 100 beats/minute. This commonly arises from a "circus rhythm" in a re-entrant pathway, most often in the atrio-ventricular node. The treatment of this re-entrant rhythm necessarily involves an interruption of the re-entrant pathway.

Vagal manoeuvres cause stimulation of the vagus nerve, which results in an atrioventricular conduction delay. The manoeuvres are most effective in a young patient, and when the patient is recumbent – so if attempted in an elderly patient who is sitting up, they are unlikely to be effective! The Valsalva manoeuvre (forced inspiration against a closed glottis) is the most reliable, but conversion to sinus rhythm is on *release* of the Valsalva, not during the manoeuvre. Alternatives are carotid sinus massage (over the carotid pulse at the level of the thyroid cartilage, on one side at a time only), eyeball pressure (but beware of contact lenses, and of producing retinal detachment), and the diving reflex (a bradycardia on diving into cold water). This latter reflex is virtually vestigial in man, but can be useful in terminating re-entrant tachycardia in small children where it is variously invoked by eating ice cream, placing a cold wet flannel over the face, or dipping the face into a basin of ice-cold water (brutal, but effective).

When the vagal manoeuvre fails the next line of treatment is adenosine, a naturally occurring purine nucleotide that is metabolised by red blood cells. Its half-life is therefore very short at ~10 seconds. It has a direct effect on the atrioventricular node, causing temporary slowing or blockade of conduction.[1] This is highly effective in treating a re-entrant tachycardia – if you like, it shuts the door in the re-entrant circuit. The short half-life of adenosine has the following implications:

- Adenosine must be given as a rapid bolus, followed by a rapid flush
- Adenosine must be given as centrally as possible (antecubital fossa is acceptable, but the back of the hand is not)

[1] DiMarco J, Sellers T, Lerman B, *et al.* Diagnostic and therapeutic use of adenosine in patients with supraventricular tachyarrhythmias. *J Am Coll Cardiol* 1985;6:417–25.

- Adenosine can be safely repeated after 2 minutes without any cumulative effects
- Adenosine is safe, even in the presence of "symptomatic" SVT (chest pain, cardiac failure, hypotension, altered level of response)
- Adenosine can be used as a diagnostic aid in broad complex tachycardia (VT will not respond; but SVT with aberrant conduction may be terminated).

The exceptions

Adenosine is contraindicated in atrial fibrillation with pre-excitation (for example, Wolff-Parkinson-White syndrome). It should not be used in sick sinus syndrome with 2nd or 3rd degree block unless a pacemaker is fitted. Adenosine can induce bronchospasm and is *relatively* contraindicated in asthmatics.

Endogenous adenosine can be responsible for clinically significant dysrhythmias in patients suffering acute myocardial infarction.[2] Bradycardia and heart block that occurs in this context and is unresponsive to conventional doses of atropine has been shown in limited practice to be responsive to a slow intravenous bolus of theophylline, 100 mg/min to a maximum of 150–250 mg.[3] Theophylline is a direct antagonist of adenosine, as are all xanthine derivatives. This is further supported by anecdotal[4] and prospective randomised controlled trial[5] evidence of successful resuscitation using aminophylline in refractory cardiac arrest with asystole.

[2] Wesley R, Lerman B, DiMarco J, Berne R, Belardinelli L. Mechanism of atropine-resistant atrioventricular block during inferior myocardial infarction: possible role of adenosine. *J Am Coll Cardiol* 1986;**8**:1232–4.
[3] Bertolet B, McMurtrie E, Hill J, Belardinelli L. Theophylline for the treatment of atrioventricular block after myocardial infarction. *Ann Intern Med* 1995;**123**:509–11.
[4] Perouansky M, Shamir M, Hershkowitz E, Donchin Y. Successful resuscitation using aminophylline in refractory cardiac arrest with asystole. *Resuscitation* 1998;**38**:39–41.
[5] Mader T, Gibson P. Adenosine receptor antagonism in refractory asystolic cardiac arrest: results of a human pilot study. *Resuscitation* 1997;**35**:3–7.

A positive pericardiocentesis only indicates there is a clot at both ends of the needle*

The reason

Needle pericardiocentesis has been recommended for the immediate management of traumatic pericardial tamponade. The rationale is that removal of a small volume of blood may restore effective cardiac output. While this can be true, the procedure may not be effective. A needle pericardiocentesis *must not delay* the definitive treatment for this condition, which is open decompression of the pericardium and direct repair of the injured muscle.

In a study of 85 patients who underwent pericardiocentesis for cardiac tamponade following trauma, there was a recurrence of tamponade with deterioration in vital signs in 35 cases[1] (and the mortality increased from 16% to 23% for those who had a recurrence of tamponade). Further, indirect evidence for a non-interventional approach pre-hospital comes from a group of "potentially salvageable" patients with penetrating cardiac trauma who either received "stabilisation" or "no stabilisation" pre-hospital. There was an 83% survival rate in those with NO stabilisation, but there were no survivors in the group who incurred a delay for intervention.[2]

Moreno and colleagues demonstrated that a tamponade following penetrating cardiac injury may have a protective effect by forestalling exsanguination.[3] Of their patients who had a tamponade, 73% survived, whereas only 11% of those with a penetrating cardiac injury, but without a tamponade, survived.

The exceptions

In 1883 Theodore Billroth wrote that, "The surgeon who should attempt to suture a wound of the heart would lose the respect of his

* This rule is attributed to Dr Ken Boffard, Principal Trauma Surgeon at Johannesburg General Hospital.

[1] Durham L, Richardson R, Wall M, *et al.* Emergency center thoracotomy: impact of prehospital resuscitation. *J Trauma* 1992;**32**:775.
[2] Gervin A, Fischer R. The importance of prompt transport in salvage of patients with penetrating heart wounds. *J Trauma* 1982;**22**:443.
[3] Moreno C, Moore EE, *et al.* Pericardial tamponade: a critical determinant for survival following penetrating cardiac wounds. *J Trauma* 1986;**26**:821.

colleagues".[4] Repeated pericardiocentesis was still being advocated as the preferred treatment in 1943.[5] In modern practice, this is not a definitive treatment option, but it does have a role in temporary stabilisation of a patient in centres not equipped to perform major operations in the emergency department.[6] If there is cardiorespiratory arrest pre-hospital following blunt cardiac injury, there is no value in pericardiocentesis or thoracotomy – the survival is 0%.[7]

A non-traumatic effusion that has developed slowly, for example as a result of infection, may have a rapid and sustained response to needle pericardiocentesis.

When it is necessary to perform the technique the standard approach is to introduce a 16–18 g long needle adjacent to the left edge of the xiphisternum, 45° below the horizontal plane, and 45° to the patient's right of the sagittal plane. The needle is gently aspirated as it is inserted. In a planned procedure, echocardiography can be used to guide the needle. A modification of this technique is to insert the needle at 45° above the horizontal plane, and to advance towards the RIGHT shoulder. The needle is then parallel rather than at right angles to the apex of the ventricle, and the possibility of myocardial injury is decreased.[8]

[4] Richardson R (ed). *The scalpel and the heart*. Scribner's: New York, 1970.
[5] Blalock A, Ravitch M. A consideration of the nonoperative treatment of cardiac tamponade resulting from wounds of the heart. *Surgery* 1943;**14**:157.
[6] Feliciano D, Moore E, Mattox K. *Trauma*, 3rd edn. Connecticut: Appleton & Lange, 1996.
[7] Mansour M, Moore EE, Moore EA, *et al*. Exigent post-injury thoracotomy – analysis of blunt vs penetrating trauma. *Surg Gynecol Obstet* 1992;**175**:97.
[8] Tate J, Horan P. Penetrating injuries of the heart. *Surg Gynecol Obstet* 1983;**157**:57.

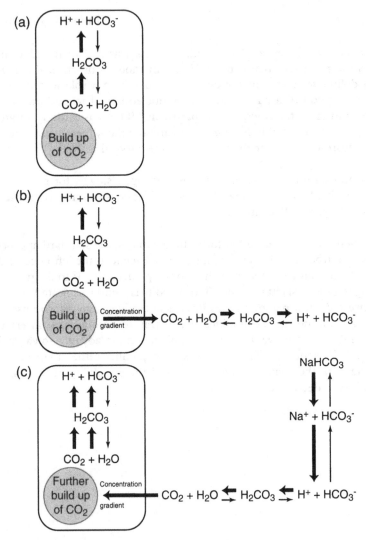

Respiratory acidosis following cardiac arrest.

(a) Intracellular respiratory acidosis after cardiorespiratory arrest.
(b) Extracellular respiratory acidosis following cardiorespiratory arrest.
(c) Worsening of intracellular acidosis with sodium bicarbonate, in the absence of effective ventilation to remove CO_2.

Ease off the base or you'll pump up the acid

The reason

Intravenous sodium bicarbonate can paradoxically increase the intracellular acidosis that occurs following cardiac arrest. To understand this consider the following pathway of events:

1 Carbon dioxide and water combine in the body to form carbonic acid, which then dissociates to form hydrogen ions and bicarbonate ions. This is represented by the equation:

$$H_2O \; + \; CO_2 \; \leftrightarrow \; H_2CO_3 \; \leftrightarrow \; H^+ \; + \; HCO_3^-$$

water · carbon dioxide · carbonic acid · hydrogen ions · bicarbonate ions

2 The direction of this equation is determined by the relative concentrations of the components at each end. If there is a high concentration of carbon dioxide the equation will be driven from left to right; if there is a high concentration of bicarbonate ions, it will be driven from right to left.

3 Following cardiac arrest there is a build up of CO_2 inside the body's cells, which results in an intracellular acidosis (the equation is driven from left to right, producing more hydrogen ions).

4 At the same time, carbon dioxide diffuses out of the cell into the vascular compartment down a concentration gradient. As the extracellular CO_2 concentration also rises, there is an extracellular acidosis.

5 When sodium bicarbonate is given intravenously, it dissociates into sodium (Na^+) and bicarbonate (HCO_3^-) ions. The extracellular equation is driven from right to left, in turn forcing CO_2 back into the cells to cause a worsening of the intracellular acidosis.

The principal treatment of acidosis following cardiac arrest is to provide effective ventilation to remove excess CO_2.

The exceptions

Cardiac arrest results in a mixed respiratory and metabolic acidosis. If the pH is <7·1 (or base excess < −10 mmol/l) after effective ventilation to remove excess CO_2 then small aliquots of intravenous sodium bicarbonate may be given, guided by repeated blood gas analysis.[1]

Sodium bicarbonate should be given early as part of the treatment for hyperkalaemia or tricyclic antidepressant poisoning, when either is a suspected cause of the cardiac arrest.

[1] Advanced Life Support Course Sub-Committee. *Advanced Life Support Course Provider Manual,* 3rd edn. London: Resuscitation Council (UK), 1998

There is no value in the emergency transportation of a corpse

The reason

Failure to respond to pre-hospital advanced cardiac life support protocols is a reliable predictor that the patient will fail to respond to resuscitative measures at the hospital.[1,2] Kellermann et al. analysed nearly 300 consecutive pre-hospital cardiac arrests where pre-hospital advanced cardiac life support measures had failed to restore a spontaneous circulation. A spontaneous circulation was restored in the emergency department in 13·3%, but only 1·6% (4 patients) survived to discharge and half of these had severe neurological impairment.[1] In a larger study of over 2300 patients where CPR was in progress on arrival at hospital, Herlitz et al. found only 28 patients (1·2%) were discharged from hospital, and only 11 (0·5%) of these had "good cerebral performance".[3]

The high speed transportation of a corpse from the scene to the hospital places the ambulance crew and other road users at unnecessary risk.[4] The cynic would say all that is achieved is a change in the geographical site of death. There is a need to identify those patients whom it is inappropriate to transport and where death can be pronounced at the scene.[5,6]

Ambulance services in the UK are increasingly issuing protocols to allow the ambulance officer to determine when not to start resuscitation. Such protocols are still of relatively low clinical impact as they are restricted to conditions where there is rigor mortis present, decapitation, or visible decomposition. Pre-hospital personnel commonly encounter terminally ill patients, and cancer is second only to

[1] Kellermann A, Staves D, Hackman B. In-hospital resuscitation following unsuccessful prehospital advanced cardiac life support: 'heroic efforts' or an exercise in futility. *Ann Emerg Med* 1988;**17**:589–94.

[2] Hodgetts T, Brown T, Hanson J, Driscoll P. Pre-hospital cardiac arrest: room for improvement. *Resuscitation* 1995;**29**:47–54.

[3] Herlitz J, Ekström L, Axelsson Å, et al. Continuation of CPR on admission to emergency department after out-of-hospital cardiac arrest. Occurrence, characteristics and outcome. *Resuscitation* 1997;**33**:223–31.

[4] Auerbach P, Morris J, Phillips J, Redinger S, Vaughn W. An analysis of ambulance accidents in Tennessee. *JAMA* 1987;**258**:1487–90.

[5] Gray W, Capone R, Most A. Unsuccessful emergency resuscitation – are continued efforts in the emergency department justified? *N Engl J Med* 1991;**325**:1393–8.

[6] Eisenberg M, Cummins R. Termination of CPR in the prehospital arena. *Ann Emerg Med* 1985;**14**:1106–7.

cardiovascular disease as the leading cause of mortality in the UK and the USA. Guidelines are needed for "do not resuscitate" orders in the pre-hospital setting, and protocols for the ambulance service when presented with such an order by a relative.[7]

The exceptions

Bonnin *et al.* concluded that resuscitation should be discontinued pre-hospital after 25 minutes of advanced cardiac life support protocols with the following exclusions, when patients should be transported to hospital:[8]

- Persistent ventricular fibrillation
- Hypothermia
- Children
- Primary cardiac arrest.

To this list it is reasonable to add persistent ventricular tachycardia, near drowning, and drug overdose.

[7] Bonnin M, Pepe P, Kimball K, Clark P. Distinct criteria for termination of resuscitation in the out-of-hospital setting. *JAMA* 1993;**270**:1457–62.

[8] American College of Emergency Physicians. Guidelines for 'do not resuscitate' orders in the prehospital setting. *Ann Emerg Med* 1988;17:1106–8.

Resuscitation is not resurrection

The reason

Resuscitation is performed by clinicians, not magicians. A successful outcome from cardiac arrest is almost always dependent on early basic life support and early defibrillation for VF or pulseless VT. Failure to achieve either of these will progressively reduce survival.

Where bystander CPR is absent, ambulance response times are slow, and advanced cardiac life support guidelines poorly followed in a prolonged resuscitation attempt at the scene, there will be no survivors leaving hospital – despite a highly trained resuscitation team within the accident and emergency department.[1] The value of transporting a corpse at high speed to hospital must then be questioned (see Rule 26). Specifically, when basic life support is delayed for more than 8–12 minutes and defibrillation is delayed more than 16 minutes, there are no survivors.[2]

The ethical decision whether to start CPR out-of-hospital can be difficult. In many aspects of medicine it is increasingly necessary to take account of the patient's wishes, but in most cases the sudden and unexpected nature of a cardiac arrest will preclude this. In Europe, and in the UK in particular, ambulance personnel are not generally empowered with the authority to decide not to begin resuscitation. Patients must be transported to hospital where a doctor can continue the resuscitation attempt or pronounce death on arrival. A study of paramedics in Oslo, who are given the power to decide whether or not to begin resuscitation, is summarised in the table below:[3]

Factors that encouraged paramedics to start resuscitation	Factors that did not influence the decision to start resuscitation
Expectations of bystanders The reputation of the emergency medical system Presence of ventricular fibrillation Pupil constriction or "normal" skin colour Arrest witnessed by paramedic The need for practice	The age of the patient alone The social status of the patient Attempted suicide

[1] Hodgetts T, Brown T, Hanson J, Driscoll P. Pre-hospital cardiac arrest: room for improvement. *Resuscitation* 1995;29:47–54.

[2] Eisenberg M, Bergner L, Hallstrom A. Cardiac resuscitation in the community: importance of rapid provision and implications for programme planning. *JAMA* 1979; 241:1905.

[3] Naess A-C, Steen E, Steen P. Ethics in treatment decisions during out-of-hospital resuscitation. *Resuscitation* 1997;33:245–56.

The exceptions

Profound hypothermia may have a cardio-protective effect and survival is recorded with delayed rescue following cold water immersion, particularly in children.[4] The characteristics of survivors are dichotomous, with either a full recovery **or** severe handicap. Of those children with a sustained return of spontaneous circulation who are admitted to hospital, a high proportion can be expected to make a full neurological recovery (86% of 188 children in one study[4]). Resuscitation attempts should not be abandoned until the child has been rewarmed (core temperature >33°C). Brain death criteria should be sought when pupil dilation persists 6 hours after rewarming.

[4] Kemp A, Sibert J. Outcome in children who nearly drown: a British Isles study. *BMJ* 1991;**302**:931–3.

Do not resuscitate to bed availability

The reason

The absence of available intensive care resources is not a reason to fail to start resuscitation, or to curtail resuscitation. This is an indication for "treat and transfer".

The exceptions

Triage is the sorting of casualties into priorities for treatment. The recognised categories are "immediate" (priority 1), "urgent" (priority 2), "delayed" (priority 3), and "dead". In a mass casualty situation, where the number of patients greatly exceeds the available resources to treat all those seriously ill or injured simultaneously, an additional triage category may be introduced – this is the "expectant" category. The principle here is *to do the most for the most*. Those who will die despite treatment receive minimal care, to allow resources to be directed towards those who are potentially salvageable.

In practice this situation is highly unlikely in a civilian "major incident", and is not known to have been used in any of the incidents (well publicised rail crashes, aircraft crashes, bombs, or crowd crushes) in the UK in the last two decades. It would be charitable to say the reason is that there are always adequate resources to treat all casualties simultaneously. However, evidence shows that triage is performed poorly at the scene of a major incident,[1,2] and it is probably more realistic to say that in many cases the "expectant" category is not even considered.

[1] Van Amerongen R, Fine J, Tunik M, Young G, Foltin G. The Avianca plane crash: an emergency medical system's response to pediatric survivors of the disaster. *Pediatr* 1993;**92**:105–10.
[2] Hodgetts T, Hall J, Maconochie I, Smart C. Paediatric triage tape. *Pre-hospital Immediate Care* 1998;**2**:155–9.

Every shroud has a silver lining

The reason

The donation of organs following death may have a profound effect on the lives of multiple recipients. The following organs may be donated post mortem:

- Heart
- Lungs
- Skin
- Cornea
- Kidneys
- Liver.

In the UK it is necessary to obtain the consent of the next of kin prior to organ harvest, even if the victim carries a "Kidney Donor" card indicating their willingness to be an organ donor. In the USA organs may be taken for donation without actively seeking consent, although any objection from the next of kin must be respected.

Any patient who is brainstem dead following traumatic head injury, subarachnoid haemorrhage, cerebral hypoxia, fat or air embolism, or drug overdose should be considered as a potential organ donor.

The exceptions

Some of the most suitable patients to be organ donors are those who die early following injury, particularly those with isolated closed head injury. It can be very difficult for staff to raise the subject of organ donation while relatives are coping with the psychological shock of the incident. This explains the very low rate of organ donation in the UK.

Specific contraindications to organ donation are serious systemic disease (diabetes, malignancy), systemic infection, or infectious disease (HIV and hepatitis B status must be negative). Age restrictions for the donor often apply, although these may vary; *for example 10–65 years for cornea, <60 years for kidney, <50 years for liver, <40 years for male heart, and <45 years for female heart.

---

* Source: Organ Donor Foundation of South Africa.

Medical emergencies

Almost anything can be done at the scene, but this does not mean that it should

The reason

The discussion between "scoop and run" versus "stay and stabilise" has been raging since the development of emergency medical care systems. There are as many proponents of advanced interventions at the scene as there are adversaries, which only emphasises that there is no clear general agreement. It is more appropriate to think in terms of a flexible spectrum of interventions, rather than an "all or nothing" approach.

In some circumstances the answer to this dilemma is becoming clearer. In the case of cardiac arrest pre-hospital, it is possible for paramedic personnel to perform the entire protocol for any rhythm. The question is, does this improve outcome over limited intervention and early movement to hospital?

In a prospective study of 502 consecutive adult patients with cardiopulmonary arrest of primary cardiac origin, Guly et al. compared the outcome from treatment by ambulance technicians or paramedics. Both were equipped with semiautomatic defibrillators. There was no significant difference in outcome between the two groups measured by a return of spontaneous circulation or survival to hospital discharge.[1] The inference is that outcome is unaffected by the advanced airway techniques and intravenous drugs that paramedics can deliver. In a follow-up study, Mitchell and Guly et al. examined the effect of full implementation of advanced skills by ambulance personnel on the outcome from pre-hospital cardiac arrest. No improvement in survival was demonstrated with more advanced pre-hospital care. In fact, 8·7% of the technician treated group survived to discharge from hospital, while 5·2% of the paramedic group survived (patients were matched for availability of bystander CPR, and for the primary presenting rhythm).[2]

[1] Guly U, Mitchell R, Cook R, Steedman D, Robertson C. Paramedics and technicians are equally successful at managing cardiac arrest outside hospital. BMJ 1995;310: 1091–4.
[2] Mitchell R, Guly U, Rainer T, Robertson C. Can the full range of paramedic skills improve survival from out of hospital cardiac arrests? J Accid Emerg Med 1997;14: 274–7.

As a further illustration, evidence shows that the insertion of a chest drain pre-hospital is associated with a high incidence of complications,[3,4] although other authors maintain that it is a safe and effective procedure in the field if the blunt dissection technique is used.[5]

The exceptions

When the pre-hospital transfer time is extended, or when further interventions *en route* will be difficult (for example, in a helicopter) then the pendulum will swing in favour of greater intervention at the scene before transport. No protocol will fit every clinical situation and the judgement relating to when it is appropriate to move a patient will be determined by the experience of the provider, and the resources available at the scene.

[3] Baldt M, Bankier A, German P, *et al.* Complications after emergency tube thoracostomy: assessment with CT. *Radiology* 1995;**195**:539–43.
[4] Peters S, Wolter D, Schultz J-H. Gefahren und Risiken der Thoraxdrainage. *Unfallchirurg* 1996;**99**:953–7.
[5] Schmidt U, Stalp M, Gerich T, Blauth M, Maull K. Chest tube decompression of blunt chest injuries by physicians in the field: effectiveness and complications. *J Trauma* 1998;**44**:98–101.

A stethoscope is no more than a badge of office

The reason

The pre-hospital environment can be noisy, and a stethoscope will not detect subtle signs. This is also true in a busy accident and emergency department. Signs that you can see and feel are often more reliable than signs you can hear. For example, the distressed, dyspnoeic patient with a unilateral hyperinflated chest (ribs splayed on the affected side), distended neck veins, and a deviated trachea away from the affected side has a tension pneumothorax. Listening for absent breath sounds is useful, but there is sufficient information to make the diagnosis already. Percussion for hyper-resonance is generally academic in the noisy pre-hospital or resuscitation environment, where a stethoscope around the neck merely acts to identify the paramedic or doctor.

As subtle signs can be easily missed in the emergency room, it is appropriate to include the chest x-ray as part of the examination of a patient who is acutely short of breath from injury or illness.

The exceptions

When the conditions do allow careful examination of the chest by auscultation, much information can be derived to localise acute changes including pneumothorax, haemothorax, consolidation, and effusion.

Can't talk, can't breathe

The reason

The inability to complete a sentence, or to count from one to ten, is a reliable clinical indicator of severe breathlessness.

With asthma indicators of a severe acute attack in adults include:

- Respiratory rate ≥25/minute
- Pulse rate ≥110/minute
- Peak expiratory flow rate ≤50% predicted.

Signs of life-threatening asthma include:

- Cyanosis
- Exhaustion
- Bradycardia
- Agitation or reduced level of response secondary to hypoxia
- Peak expiratory flow rate ≤33%
- Silent chest
- Easily palpable *pulsus paradoxus.*

A "silent chest" occurs when the bronchoconstriction is so severe that there is insufficient airflow to produce a wheeze. *Pulsus paradoxus* describes a reduction in pulse volume during inspiration (also occurs with a cardiac tamponade). Silence is not golden: in asthma it is blue!

The exceptions

A verbal response cannot be used as a guideline in infants and small children. Peak flow readings will also be unreliable in this group. Important signs of acute severe asthma in small children (≤4 years) include:

- Respiratory rate ≥50/minute
- Pulse rate ≥140/minute
- Use of accessory muscles (including intercostal muscles and diaphragm).

The life-threatening features are the same as in adults.

Principal source: British Thoracic Society. The British Guidelines on Asthma Management. *Thorax* 1997;**52**(suppl):1–21.

Beware the asthmatic with a normal pCO_2

The reason

During an episode of bronchospasm an asthmatic will hyperventilate. A consequence of hyperventilation is to "blow off" carbon dioxide. The partial pressure of carbon dioxide in the blood (pCO_2), as measured by arterial blood gases, will fall below the normal range of 4·6–6·0 kPa.

As the patient tires the pCO_2 will creep into the normal range. A normal pCO_2 in this situation is a sign of fatigue and should alert the doctor to consider elective ventilation. To wait for the pCO_2 to rise above the normal range is to invite the complications of established respiratory failure and profound hypoxia.

The exceptions

Between acute attacks of bronchospasm an asthmatic can be expected to have a normal pCO_2, in the absence of coexisting chronic lung disease.

End tidal CO_2 ($ETCO_2$) monitoring is widely used intraoperatively and can immediately detect disconnection of the tracheal tube. It can also rapidly diagnose cardiac arrest. In elective surgical procedures the $ETCO_2$ reflects the arterial pCO_2 with a deviation of 3–8 mmHg. In emergency situations $ETCO_2$ has been shown to correlate *very poorly* with arterial CO_2 concentrations,[1] and capnometry has a limited role to accurately adjust the ventilation. This can be explained by the fact that almost any degree of cardiorespiratory failure causes changes of the ventilation-perfusion ratio, impairing pulmonary CO_2 elimination. Serial arterial blood gas analysis is required to adjust ventilation parameters.

A comparison of end tidal carbon dioxide ($ETCO_2$) monitor changes with blood gas changes in common emergencies (after Feliciano et al.[2])

Problem	ETCO₂ monitor	Arterial gases
Hypoventilation	CO_2 increases	CO_2 increases
Hyperventilation	CO_2 decreases	CO_2 decreases
Cardiac output falls	CO_2 decreases	CO_2 increases
Leak in system	Nitrogen present	O_2 decreases

[1] Prause G, Hetz H, Lauda P, Pojer H, Smolle-Juettner F, Smolle JA. Comparison of the end-tidal-CO_2 documented by capnometry and the arterial pCO_2 in emergency patients. *Resuscitation* 1997;**35**:145–8.
[2] Feliciano D, Moore E, Mattox K (eds). *Trauma*, 3rd edn. Connecticut: Appleton & Lange, 1996.

The pulse oximeter measures oxygenation, not ventilation

The reason

Adequate ventilation is a combination of adequate oxygenation and adequate carbon dioxide excretion. The pulse oximeter measures the colourimetric difference between oxygenated haemoglobin and deoxygenated haemoglobin through a surface probe (nail bed, earlobe, nose) and expresses this as a percentage.

An early deterioration in ventilation may not be detected by pulse oximetry in a patient who is receiving high concentration oxygen. The pulse oximeter may continue to register "100%" saturation, despite a rise in the carbon dioxide concentration.

The exceptions

In a patient breathing air, a fall in oxygen saturation measured by pulse oximetry is a reliable sign of deteriorating ventilation. However, this is not a linear but a sigmoidal ("S"-shaped) relationship – so that a small initial fall in percentage oxygen saturation indicates a significant fall in the partial pressure of oxygen.

One study of children less than two years old with lower respiratory infections evaluated the concordance of pulse oximetry readings with clinical signs. The authors concluded that there was a poor correlation and oximetry should be performed in all these patients because of the poor reliability of clinical signs.[1]

A separate study of 2127 "non-critical" children presenting to a paediatric emergency department compared physicians' evaluations of children before and after seeing the results of pulse oximetry. In 305 children oxygen saturation values were <95% on air, and physicians adjusted their evaluations in 95 of these children.[2] It is a simple and non-invasive test in this group of patients and is arguably a "fifth vital sign" (respiratory rate, pulse, blood pressure, temperature, oximetry).

Conversely, a normal oxygen saturation measured by pulse oximetry (SpO_2) must not preclude supplemental oxygen in a critically ill patient.

[1] Wang E, Milner R, Navas L, Maj H. Observer agreement for respiratory signs and oximetry in infants hospitalized with lower respiratory infections. *Am Rev Respir Dis* 1992;**145**:106–9.
[2] Mower W. Pulse oximetry as a fifth pediatric vital sign. *Pediatr* 1997;**99**:681–6.

How does pulse oximetry work?

Pulse oximetry measures oxygen saturation of haemoglobin under ideal conditions. Two wavelengths of light are emitted – oxyhaemoglobin absorbs the near infra-red band (940 nm) and deoxygenated haemoglobin absorbs the red band (660 nm). Oxygen saturation is determined by measuring the ratio of red *vs* near infra-red light entering the detector.

Recognised pitfalls

- The pulse oximeter does not distinguish carboxyhaemoglobin. The true oxygen saturation may be as little as half that reflected by the oximeter[3]
- Methaemoglobin forces the saturation towards 85%[4]
- False readings are also produced by extraneous light, dyes (particularly methylene blue), and blue or green nail polish[5]
- The majority of oximeters are tested for accuracy only as low as 70% saturation, which represents the lower limit of tolerable hypoxia (approximates to a paO_2 of 5 kPa). Above 70% saturation, the error is $\pm 2\%$.[6]

[3] Barker S, Tremper K. The effect of carbon monoxide inhalation on pulse oximeter signal detection. *Anesthesiology* 1988;**66**:677.
[4] Barker S, Tremper K, Hyatt J, *et al.* Effects of methaemoglobinaemia on pulse oximetry and mixed venous oximetry. *Anesthesiology* 1988;**70**:112.
[5] Feliciano D, Moore E, Mattox K (eds). *Trauma*, 3rd edn. Connecticut: Appleton & Lange, 1996.
[6] Healy T, Cohen P (eds). *A practice of anaesthesia*, 6th edn. London: Edward Arnold, 1995.

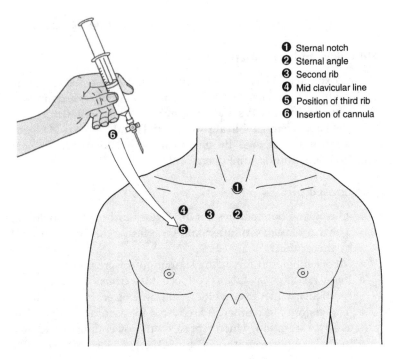

1 Sternal notch
2 Sternal angle
3 Second rib
4 Mid clavicular line
5 Position of third rib
6 Insertion of cannula

Landmarks for decompressing a tension pneumothorax.

(a) Place your finger in the sternal notch and trace down the sternum until you reach the sternal angle (*Angle of Louis*)
(b) Move laterally onto the second rib and as far as the mid-clavicular line
(c) Go below the second rib, and insert the cannula just above the third rib (thereby avoiding the neurovascular bundle that runs along the inferior aspect of each rib)

In a ventilation crisis, to cope remember DOPE

The reason

A sudden deterioration in a patient's condition whilst providing ventilation (via an automatic ventilator, or via a bag-valve system) requires a systematic approach to eliminate the most likely causes.

D	Displaced tube	Check for equal breath sounds, and observe for equal chest movement. Listen over the epigastrium to identify accidental oesophageal intubation. Remember, it is not negligent to intubate the oesophagus, only to fail to recognise it (see *Trauma Rules*, Rule 9).[1]
O	Oxygen	Check that the oxygen source has not run out. A Waters' circuit cannot function without an oxygen source (see Rule 15). Has the oxygen tubing become kinked (e.g. under the wheel of the trolley)? Are you inadvertently ventilating from piped air, rather than piped oxygen?
P	Pneumothorax	Has a pneumothorax developed? Is it a *tension* pneumothorax, requiring immediate needle decompression (see Rule 38, and figure opposite)?
E	Equipment failure	If you are using a ventilator, immediately disconnect and start ventilation with a bag-valve-mask apparatus. If you are using a bag-valve-mask, change your system and reassess (the system may be faulty, or it may have been reassembled incorrectly after cleaning).

The exceptions

Although the components of this rule hold true, some would argue that the first action would be to check for equipment failure ("EDOP").

[1] Hodgetts T, Deane S, Gunning K. *Trauma Rules*. London: BMJ Publishing Group, 1997.

The patient who refuses oxygen is often hypoxic

The reason

Hypoxia will produce a predictable alteration in response through agitation, confusion, combativeness, and coma. The patient who resists the oxygen mask being placed on their face may simply be uncooperative, but should be presumed to be hypoxic.

A hypoxic patient who becomes calm should not be presumed to be improving, as agitation will succumb to coma with progressive hypoxia. It is important not only to monitor the state of agitation, but to objectively monitor the level of response by repeated Glasgow Coma Scale assessments, and to monitor improvements in oxygenation by continuous pulse oximetry and serial blood gas measurements (but, see Rule 34).

The exceptions

There is no significant exception to this rule.

When the GCS is eight, proceed now to intubate

The reason

The Glasgow Coma Scale (GCS) is an objective reproducible measure of brain function. The maximum score is 15, and the minimum score is 3. A score of 8 or less is the definition of "coma". Endotracheal intubation is required in these circumstances principally to protect the airway from aspiration of gastric contents, but with the additional requirement of improving inadequate ventilation (optimising oxygenation, and avoiding hypercarbia with the secondary effect of cerebral vasodilatation).

The exceptions

In general terms a patient will not die from lack of intubation, but from lack of oxygenation (see *Trauma Rules*, Rule 9). If the skills to perform intubation are unavailable, simple airway manoeuvres and adjuncts will usually be adequate to sustain the patient. However, early elective intubation is the best clinical practice.

If you cannot decompress a tension, think laterally and go laterally

The reason

The common teaching for the management of a tension pneumothorax is immediate needle decompression with a 3–6 cm long wide-bore peripheral intravenous cannula in the second intercostal space, mid-clavicular line.[1]

This will fail to release the air under tension if the thickness of the chest wall is greater than the length of the needle. This can be anticipated in the muscular adult male, the obese, or the patient with generalised oedema. In the UK the most frequent cannula length is 4·5 cm. In an ultrasound study of 54 consecutive adults aged 18–55 years the chest wall diameter at the site of insertion for a needle thoracocentesis was >4·5 cm in 4%.[2]

The chest wall is thinner in the mid-axillary line. When you are certain of the diagnosis and conventional needle thoracocentesis fails, *think laterally and go laterally.* The alternative is to proceed immediately to a tube thoracostomy (chest drain).

An additional reason for delayed failure is that the tip of the cannula may just reach the pleural space while pressure is applied during insertion, but on release of pressure the cannula backs out of the pleural space as the skin of the chest wall regains its shape.[3]

The exceptions

Before going laterally remove the metal introducer needle. It is possible that there is a plug (of skin, fat, or muscle) inside this needle, and the cannula will drain air once the introducer is removed.

[1] American College of Surgeons, Committee on Trauma. *Advanced Trauma Life Support Course Manual.* Washington DC: ACS, 1993.

[2] Britten S, Palmer S, Snow T. Needle thoracocentesis in tension pneumothorax: insufficient cannula length and potential failure. *Injury* 1996;27:321–2.

[3] Britten S, Palmer S. Chest wall thickness may limit adequate drainage of tension pneumothorax by needle thoracocentesis. *J Accid Emerg Med* 1996;13:426–7.

Needle thoracocentesis may also be unsuccessful if the tension pneumothorax is localised or loculated,[4] or if the air leak is greater than the rate of drainage from the needle.[5]

The chest is not the only body cavity that can contain air under tension. Air under tension in the abdomen (tension pneumoperitoneum) has been reported secondary to the following:

- Recent bowel surgery and positive pressure ventilation[6]
- Leakage through alveolar walls during high pressure ventilation, then tracking along perivascular sheaths to the mediastinum, and via the diaphragmatic openings to the retroperitoneal space and peritoneum[7]
- Congenital and acquired diaphragmatic defects[8]
- Gas forming organisms[9]
- Cardiopulmonary resuscitation.[10]

The increase in intra-abdominal pressure may inhibit ventilation, compress the inferior vena cava, and even compress the abdominal aorta.[11] Consideration should be given to decompressing the peritoneal cavity with a large bore cannula.

[4] Mines D, Abbuhl S. Needle thoracostomy fails to detect a fatal tension pneumothorax. *Ann Emerg Med* 1993;**22**:133.

[5] Conces D, Tarver R, Gray W, *et al.* Treatment of pneumothoraces utilising small caliber chest tubes. *Chest* 1988;**94**:55.

[6] Roberts R, Blake B, Bruggeman G. Tension pneumoperitoneum – a cause of ventilatory obstruction. *Anesthesiology* 1981;**55**:326–7.

[7] Karlowicz M. Pneumoretroperitoneum and perirenal air associated with tension pneumothorax. *Am J Perinatol* 1994;**11**:63–4.

[8] Burdett-Smith P, Jaffey L. Tension pneumoperitoneum. *J Accid Emerg Med* 1996;**13**:220–1.

[9] Falkenburg C. Ein Fall von Gasansammlung in der freien Bauch-Hohle. *Dtsch Z Chir* 1913;**124**:130–6.

[10] Cameron P, Rosengarten P, Johnson W, Dziukas L. Tension pneumoperitoneum after cardiopulmonary resuscitation. *MJA* 1991;**155**:44–7.

[11] Olinde A, Carpenter D, Maher J. Tension pneumoperitoneum. *Arch Surg* 1983;**118**:1347–50.

Head injuries cause fits and fits cause head injuries

The reason

This is a fitting palindrome!

Trauma is the commonest cause of death from 1–35 years, and head injuries are the leading cause of mortality in those who survive to reach hospital. Direct brain injury is associated with secondary convulsions. On the other hand, a convulsion in a patient with an epileptic tendency may result in secondary injury sustained in, for example, a fall or a vehicle accident.

Many neurosurgeons will prescribe prophylactic anticonvulsants to a patient who has suffered a closed head injury. For those patients who do suffer post-traumatic seizures, treatment is commonly continued for at least 1 year. The duration of treatment for those who do not suffer a seizure has been somewhat arbitrary, but treatment beyond 8 days post-injury has not been shown to significantly reduce the incidence of seizures.[1]

The exceptions

There may be other causes of a loss of consciousness that results in a secondary head injury, with or without associated convulsions – for example, a vaso-vagal episode (faint), a cardiac dysrhythmia, or a cerebrovascular accident.

Hypoglycaemia may cause convulsions *per se*. Hypoglycaemia may be both the cause of an accident with a resulting head injury, or it may be a consequence of any severe injury (it is a common metabolic derangement in injured children, see Rule 56).

Alcohol may cause injuries which may cause fits; alcohol may cause hypoglycaemia which may cause fits, or injuries, or both; fits or injuries may aggravate alcohol-induced hypoglycaemia.

---

[1] Temkin N, Dikmen S, Wilensky A. A randomized, double-blind study of phenytoin for the prevention of post-traumatic seizures. *N Engl J Med* 1990;**323**:497.

Alcohol is not a cause of unconsciousness

The reason

Alcohol intoxication makes a person more likely to fall and injure themselves, not less likely. It is a dangerous (although frequent) presumption that a patient who is unresponsive or combative and who smells of alcohol is drunk. If head injury cannot be excluded from the history, or there are signs of head injury on examination, then it must be anticipated that the cause for altered response is brain injury. This will often require urgent evaluation by CT scanning.

The exceptions

Alcohol taken in excess can, of course, produce a profound reduction in the level of response. But this is a diagnosis of exclusion. The causes of unconsciousness can be remembered as "vowels and FITS":

A Alcohol
E Epilepsy
I Insulin (excess – hypoglycaemia; deficiency – hyperglycaemia)
O Overdose
U Uraemia

F Fever/Functional
I Infection/Ischaemia
T Trauma/Tumour
S Stroke/Shock

Pupils, pin-pricks, pulses

The reason

Pupil changes, needle track marks, and cardiac dysrhythmias are useful diagnostic indicators that the cause of unconsciousness is a drug overdose.

Pupils

Constricted pupils	Think of overdose with opiates (morphine, diamorphine [heroin], methadone); but pupil constriction will also occur with organophosphates (see Rule 42).
Dilated pupils	Think of tricyclic antidepressants and amphetamines (including Ecstasy).

Pin-pricks

Virtually anything can be injected, but common substances include morphine and diamorphine. Adverse reactions may be related to impurities with which the substance has been "cut" (mixed).

Pulses

Tachycardia	Think of tricyclic antidepressants (sinus tachycardia, SVT, fast atrial fibrillation and VT), and amphetamines (sinus tachycardia, SVT).
Bradycardia	Think of β-blockers and calcium channel blockers (taken by "ravers" to counter the effects of the amphetamines).

Ecstasy (MDMA or 3,4-methylenedioxymethamphetamine) is associated with severe and fatal reactions including hyperthermia, seizures, hypertensive crises, disseminated intravascular coagulopathy, rhabdomyolysis, hepatic toxicity, cerebrovascular accidents, spontaneous pneumomediastinum, and psychiatric disturbances.[1-3] The incidence of abuse is increasing in the UK and the USA.[4]

[1] Mallick A, Bodenham A. MDMA induced hyperthermia: a survivor with an initial body temperature of 42.9°C. *J Accid Emerg Med* 1997;**14**:336–8.
[2] Henry J, Jeffreys K, Dawling S. Toxicity and deaths from 3,4-methylenedioxy-methamphetamine ("ecstasy"). *Lancet* 1992;**340**:384–7.
[3] O'Connor B. Hazards associated with the recreational drug "ecstasy". *Br J Hosp Med* 1994;**52**:507–14.
[4] Cuomo M, Dyment P, Gammino V. Increasing use of "Ecstasy" (MDMA) and other hallucinogens on a college campus. *J Am Coll Health* 1994;**42**:271–4.

The exceptions

Don't forget that dilated pupils can indicate trauma, particularly in the unresponsive patient with unilateral pupil changes. Pin-pricks will not be a useful diagnostic aid if the patient has inhaled (smoked/ snorted) the drug. Spontaneous pneumomediastinum reported with Ecstasy has also been seen in conjunction with a number of other recreational drugs including inhalation of marijuana, cocaine, and alkaloid cocaine ("crack").

Rule 42

Organophosphate poisoning produces excess SLUDGE

The reason

Organophosphate pesticides are used extensively across the world. Annually there are an estimated 3 million cases of poisoning and about 40 000 deaths.[1] These substances also form the basis of a series of chemical warfare agents, one of which (sarin) has been implicated in terrorist attacks by the Aum Shinrikyo cult in Tokyo in 1995, where 12 died and 5500 were poisoned. Organophosphates can be inhaled, or absorbed through the skin; the lethal dose of sarin is just 0·01 mg/kg, which is less than a pin-prick sized droplet. Sarin was first produced in Germany in 1938 by the agrochemical industry,[2] and remains simple to manufacture; details of the process are, disturbingly, available on the Internet. Another derivative, tabun, was widely used by Iraq in the war against Iran between 1984 and 1988.

Organophosphates act by binding to the enzyme cholinesterase, which is required to break down acetylcholine. The result is persistent post-synaptic receptor stimulation, with side effects reflecting the potentiated action of acetylcholine. These can be remembered as "SLUDGE":

S	Salivation
L	Lacrimation
U	Urination
D	Defaecation
G	Gut cramps
E	Emesis

Decontamination is essential. It is achieved by removing the patient's clothes and washing with a detergent and bleach solution.[3] (Fuller's earth must not be placed in a wound because of its cytotoxic effects.[4]) The clothes should be sealed in a thick transparent plastic bag to prevent "off gassing"; a transparent bag is needed so it does not have

[1] Volans A. Sarin: guidelines on the management of victims of a nerve gas attack. *J Accid Emerg Med* 1996;**13**:202–6.
[2] Minton N, Murray V. A review of organophosphate poisoning. *Med Toxicol* 1988;**3**: 350–75.
[3] Morgan-Jones D, Hodgetts T. Sarin. *J Accid Emerg Med* 1996;**13**:431–3.
[4] Cooper G, Ryan J, Galbraith K. The surgical management in war of penetrating wounds contaminated with chemical warfare agents. *J R Army Med Corps* 1994;**140**: 113–8.

to be opened again to see the contents! Treatment involves repeated doses of atropine (principally to reverse salivation, bronchospasm, and bronchorrhoea) in total doses greatly in excess of the usual 3 mg maximal "full atropinisation" dose.[5] Oximes are used concurrently with atropine (for example, pralidoxime mesylate) to reactivate the cholinesterase enzyme. If this is not achieved within 24 hours the enzyme prematurely "ages" and further recovery is dependent on enzyme regeneration, which may take several weeks. Reports from the Iran–Iraq war stated that the aggressive use of atropine in the first 20–30 minutes together with oximes led to a rapid recovery from even the most severe poisoning.[3] Benzodiazepines are used to combat the associated anxiety, and for the symptomatic treatment of convulsions. Current military first aid treatment is with a combination of atropine 2 mg, pralidoxime mesylate 500 mg, and avizafone 10 mg (equivalent to 5 mg diazepam) self-administered via an intramuscular injection (spring-loaded pen device).[3]

The exceptions

Early signs of organophosphate poisoning are pupil constriction, blurred vision, and headache. These are present with sub-lethal exposure doses of vapour, and can be expected in a high proportion of hospital carers – up to 20%[6] – when there are inadequate decontamination facilities and personal protective equipment at the hospital.

[5] Suzuki T, Morita H, Ono K, *et al.* Sarin poisoning in the Tokyo subway. *Lancet* 1995; **345**:980–1.
[6] Jamal G. Long term neurotoxic effects of organophosphate compounds. *Adverse Drug React Toxicol Rev* 1995;14:85–99.

Pale and sweaty with wheeze, think cardiac disease

The reason

Acute left ventricular failure will produce severe shortness of breath, with signs of pulmonary oedema that may include wheeze audible with a stethoscope ("cardiac asthma"). These patients will characteristically be pale and sweaty.

Alternatively, acute bronchoconstriction (asthma, or exacerbation of chronic obstructive pulmonary disease) characteristically produces a patient who is short of breath, who breathes with the accessory muscles of respiration (sternomastoids; adopting the "tripod" hand position), and who purses their lips in expiration to maintain positive end expiratory pressure.

The exceptions

A patient can have concomitant obstructive airways disease and ischaemic heart disease, which may cause difficulty with the clinical differentiation of the cause of the wheeze.

Minutes equals myocardium

The reason

The benefits of thrombolytic therapy are directly related to the time from the onset of the myocardial infarction to the administration of the treatment. If given within the first hour of symptoms, thrombolysis can save up to 35 lives per 1000 treated patients.[1]

The value of giving pre-hospital thrombolysis has been shown in the GREAT study, when administered by general practitioners in remote areas.[2] The European Myocardial Infarction Project (EMIP) showed a 16% reduction in short-term cardiac mortality, with an overall reduction in mortality of 13%. This represented 15 lives saved for every 1000 patients who received pre-hospital thrombolysis.[3]

In the absence of an integrated pre-hospital system for the delivery of thrombolysis in the UK, a target of 30 minutes from time of arrival in the accident and emergency department to the start of a thrombolytic infusion has become standard practice. This is a difficult and often unrealistic target. Repeated studies have shown that the "door-to-needle" time may average more than one hour.[4-6] Audit is important within a hospital to identify the reasons for delay locally, to educate staff, and to implement measures to reduce the door-to-needle time. Such an approach has been widely reported to improve

[1] Fibrinolytic Trialists Therapy Collaborative Group. Indications for fibrinolytic therapy in suspected acute myocardial infarction: collaborative overview of early mortality and major morbidity results from all randomised trials of over 1000 patients. *Lancet* 1994;**343**:311–22.

[2] The GREAT Group. Feasibility, safety and efficacy of domiciliary thrombolysis by general practitioners: Grampian Region early anistreplase trial. *BMJ* 1992;**305**:548–53.

[3] Leizorovicz A, Boissel J, Julian D, Castaigne A, Haugh M, The European Myocardial Infarction Project Group. Prehospital thrombolytic therapy in patients with suspected myocardial infarction. *N Engl J Med* 1993;**329**:383–9.

[4] Birkhead J. Time delays in provision of thrombolytic treatment in six district hospitals. *BMJ* 1992;**305**:445–8.

[5] Kereiakes A, Weaver W, Anderson J, *et al.* Time delays in the diagnosis and treatment of acute myocardial infarction: a tale of eight cities. Report from the Pre-hospital Study Group and Cincinnati Heart Project. *Am Heart J* 1990;**120**:773–80.

[6] Sharkey S, Brunette D, Ruiz E, *et al.* An analysis of the time delays preceding thrombolysis for acute myocardial infarction. *JAMA* 1989;**262**:3171–4.

performance.[7,8] Significant factors associated with an increased delay in receiving thrombolysis have been found to be:[9]

- Incorrect triage (chest pain not given a high enough priority on arrival)
- Initial assessment by a junior doctor (with consequent incorrect or delayed diagnosis)
- Atypical presenting history of myocardial infarction
- Degrees of ST elevation less than the accepted criteria for starting treatment (1 mm or more in two or more limb leads, and 2 mm or more in two contiguous chest leads).

In patients with an equivocal ECG it is appropriate to repeat the ECG every 15–30 minutes until there are diagnostic changes.[6] The relationship between diagnostic ECG changes and hospital delay is emphasised in one study.[10] Clear guidelines are required for the management of these patients,[11,12] and it is essential that the same benchmarks are used when comparing the results of different hospitals with different patient profiles.[9]

A "fast track" policy to the coronary care unit via the accident and emergency (A&E) department has been suggested to improve the door-to-needle time. The evidence does not support this, and reveals an additional appreciable delay.[6,9,13] However, when the facility for thrombolysis does *not* exist in A&E then direct admission by the ambulance service to the coronary care unit will reduce the delay.[14]

[7] MacCallum A, Stafford P, Jones C, *et al.* Reduction of in-hospital time to thrombolytic therapy by audit of policy guidelines. *Eur Heart J* 1990;**11**(Suppl F):48–52.

[8] Porter G, Doughty R, Gamble G, Sharpe N. Thrombolysis in acute myocardial infarction: reducing in-hospital treatment delay. *N Z Med J* 1995;**108**:253–4.

[9] Palmer D, Cox C, Dear K, Leitch J. Factors associated with delay in giving thrombolytic therapy after arrival at hospital. *MJA* 1998;**168**:111–4.

[10] Sharkey S, Berger C, Brunette D, Henry T. Impact of the electrocardiogram on delivery of thrombolytic therapy for acute myocardial infarction. *Am J Cardiol* 1994;**73**:550–3.

[11] Weston C, Penny W, Julian D. Guidelines for the early management of patients with myocardial infarction. *BMJ* 1994;**308**:767–71.

[12] The Emergency Cardiac Care Coalition. Recommendations for ensuring early thrombolytic therapy for acute myocardial infarction. *Can Med Assoc J* 1996;**154**:483–7.

[13] Parry G, Wrightson W, Hood L, *et al.* Delays to thrombolysis in the treatment of myocardial infarction. *J R Coll Physicians Lond* 1993;**27**:19–23.

[14] Banerjee S, Rhoden W. Fast-tracking of myocardial infarction by paramedics. *J R Coll Physicians Lond* 1998;**32**:36–8.

There is generally a requirement in this case for the paramedic to perform a 12-lead ECG and make a provisional diagnosis of myocardial infarction, although local policy may allow direct referral to CCU based on clinical assessment alone.

The exceptions

There is a preoccupation with the door-to-needle time. The most important factors that delay administration of thrombolysis is the time taken by patients before deciding to seek help[9,15,16] and the delay in decision-making by the general practitioner. In one study of 257 proven infarcts attended at home by general practitioners in the Netherlands, 50% took more than 82 minutes before sending the patient to hospital.[17] When assessing performance in the treatment of acute myocardial infarction it is important to also consider the *pain-to-needle* time.

[15] Leitch J, Birbara T, Freedman B, *et al.* Factors influencing the time from onset of chest pain to arrival at hospital. *Med J Aust* 1997;**166**:233–6.
[16] Gurwitz J, McLaughlin T, Willison D, *et al.* Delayed hospital presentation in patients who have had acute myocardial infarction. *Ann Intern Med* 1997;**126**:593–9.
[17] Bleeker J, Simoons M, Erdman R, *et al.* Patient and doctor delay in acute myocardial infarction: a study in Rotterdam, The Netherlands. *Brit J Gen Pract* 1995;**45**:181–4.

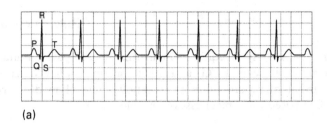

(a)

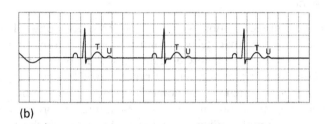

(b)

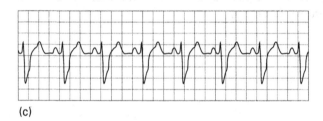

(c)

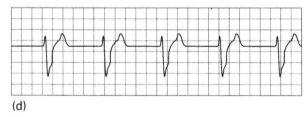

(d)

ECG characteristics of serum potassium derangement.

(a) Normal ECG
(b) Hypokalaemic ECG: note the small T wave and the prominent
    U wave (upward deflection after the T wave)
(c) Hyperkalaemic ECG, mild: note the prominent T wave
(d) Hyperkalaemic ECG, severe: note the tented T wave, absent
    P wave, bradycardia, and broad bizarre QRS complexes

No pot no T

The reason

The size of the T wave seen on the ECG is correlated with the serum potassium. Hyperkalaemia is characterised by a tall, tented T wave, whereas hypokalaemia is characterised by a small T wave.

Hypokalaemia is also characterised by a prominent U wave, a further upward deflection after the T wave (generally, U waves are positive in the leads in which T waves are normally positive). Hyperkalaemia may produce bradycardia and broad bizarre QRS complexes, with absent P waves.

The exceptions

Small ECG complexes, and hence small T waves, are also seen in hypothermia, hypothyroidism, and pericardial effusion.

The T wave is often flattened or inverted in myocardial ischaemia, hypertensive heart disease, aortic valve disease, and myocarditis (plus other less common conditions).

Ultra-early ECG signs of a myocardial infarction can be "hyperacute" (pointed) T waves in the corresponding leads, and ST segment depression representing myocardial ischaemia prior to infarction (although ST segment depression is not specific to myocardial ischaemia).

Do not be shocked when the IM route fails

The reason

Shock is defined as inadequate tissue oxygenation. This is a result of inadequate tissue perfusion. Drugs given by the intramuscular (IM) route will not be reliably absorbed if the patient is shocked. A prime example is the administration of opiate analgesics. Inadequate pain relief because of poor absorption may result in repeated doses being given. If the shocked state is suddenly reversed (for example, with restoration of circulating volume following intravenous fluid administration), toxic concentrations enter the circulation with consequent suppression of ventilation.

The intramuscular route is contraindicated in a shocked patient. The intravenous route (or intraosseous route) should be used for drug administration in this circumstance.

The exceptions

Intramuscular morphine is available to British soldiers on the battlefield to administer to wounded comrades. The use of this drug follows a strict protocol that limits the dose to 10 mg, repeated once only if necessary after 30 minutes.[1]

The Chief Medical Officer for England and Wales recommends the use of intramuscular penicillin if a general practitioner suspects meningococcal meningitis or septicaemia.[2] This has been shown to reduce mortality by over 50% in those septicaemic patients who are shocked[3] (see Rule 58).

[1] Battlefield First Aid – Aide Memoire. Army Code 71638. Crown Copyright 1998.
[2] Calman K. Meningococcal infection: meningitis and septicaemia. London: Department of Health PL/CMO(94)2, 1994.
[3] Cartwright K, Reilly S, White D, Stuart J. Early treatment with parenteral penicillin in meningococcal disease. *BMJ* 1992;305:143–52.

Avoid colloid in the critically ill: reach for the Ringer's

The reason

Recent controversial research has identified that mortality is increased when colloids are used in the resuscitation of the critically ill. A systematic review of randomised controlled trials that compared colloids with crystalloids identified that there was a 4% absolute increased mortality for those patients receiving colloid.[1] The authors recognised the limitations of the study in that the type of colloid or crystalloid varied, the concentration varied, and the protocol to determine the amount of fluid given varied. It was concluded, however, that this would affect only the size of the effect, rather than its direction and there was no indication for the continued use of colloids except for a randomised controlled trial.

This study has met with a wave of clinical criticism. Despite this, Offringa concluded that the review was scientifically sound, although he stated that beneficial effects of albumin in certain patients may have been obscured in the analysis and could not be totally excluded.[2] Supportive evidence has come from the Cochrane Injuries Group Albumin Reviewers who conclude from an independent systematic review of the value of albumin in the critically ill that, *"There is no evidence that albumin administration reduces mortality in critically ill patients with hypovolaemia, burns, or hypoalbuminaemia and a strong suggestion that it may increase mortality"*.[3]

There are a number of mechanisms that may explain why albumin may worsen the condition of the critically ill patient:

- Rapid infusion of 20% albumin leads to pulmonary oedema (baboon model in haemorrhagic shock)[4]

---

[1] Schierhout G, Roberts I. Fluid resuscitation with colloid or crystalloid solutions in critically ill patients: a systematic review of randomised trials. *BMJ* 1998;**316**:961–4.
[2] Offringa M. Excess mortality after human albumin administration in critically ill patients. *BMJ* 1998;**317**:223–4.
[3] Cochrane Injuries Group Albumin Reviewers. Human albumin administration in critically ill patients: a systematic review of randomised controlled trials. *BMJ* 1998; **317**:235–40.
[4] Moss G, Das Gupta T, Brinkman R, Sehgal L, Newsom B. Changes in lung ultrastructure following heterologous and homologous serum albumin infusion in the treatment of haemorrhagic shock. *Ann Surg* 1979;**189**:236–42.

- Albumin and water passing across "leaky" capillaries (for example, burns patients or septic patients) may cause or worsen pulmonary oedema and compromises tissue oxygenation (every 1 g of albumin that leaks from capillary to interstitium is accompanied by 18 g of water)
- Antihaemostatic and platelet lowering properties of albumin may increase blood loss in post-surgery trauma patients[5]
- Albumin in hypovolaemic shock may impair sodium and water excretion and worsen renal failure.[6]

The exceptions

New synthetic high molecular weight colloids (hydroxyethyl starches) have not been included in the systematic review analyses. These are known to have a longer plasma half-life than albumin (up to 48 hours) and when compared to albumin have been shown to be beneficial in terms of haemodynamic variables, oxygen delivery, and non-specific inhibition of the acute inflammatory response.[7]

[5] Johnson S, Lucas C, Gerrick S, Ledgerwood A, Higgins R. Altered coagulation after albumin supplements for treatment of oligaemic shock. *Arch Surg* 1979;**114**:379–83.
[6] Moon M, Lucas C, Ledgerwood A, Kosinski J. Free water clearance after supplemental albumin resuscitation for shock. *Circ Shock* 1989;**28**:1–8.
[7] Gosling P. Newer synthetic colloids should not be abandoned. *BMJ* 1998;**317**:277.

CT and LP have no place in MD

The reason

The diagnosis of meningococcal disease (MD) is principally a clinical one. The management when MD is suspected is to give immediate parenteral broad spectrum antibiotics (intravenous, intraosseous – see Rule 55, or intramuscular), and supportive therapy (see Rule 58).[1] In meningococcal septicaemia the major threat to life is shock, although severe lung injury is also common. Treatment therefore involves large volumes of fluid (see Rule 47) and inotropic support, with a low threshold for intubation and ventilation. Pulmonary oedema can be anticipated in septicaemic patients who require more than 40 ml/kg fluid resuscitation, and this is the watershed for elective intubation. It is also the milestone for starting dobutamine +/- dopamine as inotropes. In meningococcal meningitis a sudden and potentially catastrophic rise in intracranial pressure is sometimes seen that requires intubation, hyperventilation, mannitol, and discussion with an intensive care unit.

None of this initial management is dependent on the results of two time-consuming and potentially dangerous investigations – lumbar puncture (LP) and CT scan. Microscopy of cerebrospinal fluid (CSF) taken at lumbar puncture will confirm the diagnosis of bacterial meningitis (and intracellular Gram-negative diplococci will confirm it as meningococcal meningitis). It is a potentially lethal intervention if performed when there is raised intracranial pressure (coma, hypertension, bradycardia, pupil changes). Lumbar puncture will rarely help the diagnosis in the septicaemic patient as the CSF is frequently sterile.

There is a danger of laypersons, media, and health workers collectively referring to the spectrum of the disease as "meningitis". Those with isolated septicaemia have a rash, but do not have photophobia and neck stiffness, yet their mortality is very high (see Rule 58).

CT scanning will neither help the diagnosis nor alter the management.

---

[1] Hodgetts T, Brett A, Castle N. The early management of meningococcal disease. *J Accid Emerg Med* 1998;**15**:72–6.

The exceptions

When a lumbar puncture can be performed expeditiously in a patient with suspected meningitis, without unduly delaying antibiotic treatment, it can greatly contribute to an accurate early diagnosis. In particular, it may differentiate bacterial from viral meningitis (which will invariably respond conservatively), and can identify unusual organisms which require specific antibiotic combinations (for example, tuberculous meningitis).

In suspected cases of meningococcal septicaemia or meningitis, it is important to take blood cultures at hospital prior to antibiotics if possible. Where antibiotics have been given pre-hospital, alternative methods of diagnosis can be utilised. Bacteriological diagnosis can be made from a throat swab, rash aspirate, serodiagnosis, and polymerase chain reaction.

Paediatric resuscitation

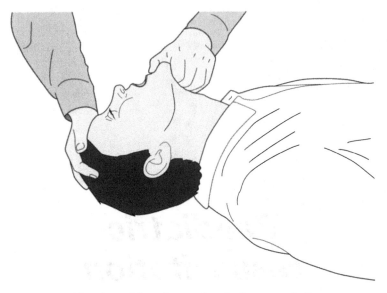

Head position for optimal airway, adult.

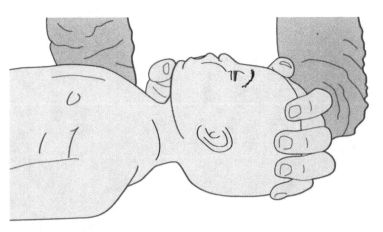

Head position for optimal airway, infant.

Babies are born with an integral pillow

The reason

The optimal head position to maintain the upper airway in an adult is with the neck flexed and the head extended as if "sniffing the morning air". As infants have a prominent occiput the neck is naturally forced into flexion when recumbent. To achieve the optimum position it is only necessary to bring the face into a plane parallel with the flat surface on which the infant is lying. Indeed to overextend the head may result in a paradoxical compromise of the airway.

The exceptions

An anencephalic child is born with the posterior of the head flattened and the brain exposed (there is complete failure of closure of the anterior neural tube). There is 100% neonatal mortality and resuscitative intervention is inappropriate.[1]

Premature closure of the cranial sutures (craniosynostosis) results in malformations of the skull, for example scaphocephaly (boat-shaped skull), acrocephaly (tower skull), and plagiocephaly (asymmetric skull).[2] These abnormalities may affect the optimal head position for the infant.

[1] Seidel H, Rosenstein B, Pathak A. Primary care of the newborn. St Louis: Mosby Year Book, 1993.
[2] Langman J. *Medical embryology*, 4th edn. Baltimore: Wiliams & Wilkins, 1982.

Rule 50

Pff–Pff–Pff–Help–Help–Help

The reason

The *pff–pff–pff* noise heard during a paediatric resuscitation attempt is air hissing through the pressure release valve built into a paediatric bag-valve-mask. This valve is designed to prevent pulmonary barotrauma.

The noise represents ineffective ventilation, as the tidal volume is being vented. The explanations are:

1 An obstructed airway secondary to poor head position (overflexed, or over-extended). The correct airway position for an infant is with the face parallel with the firm surface on which the infant is lying.
2 A rapid respiratory rate leading to raised inspiratory pressure. Here the anxiety of the inexperienced operator is the cause of overzealous compression of the bag – *it is a cry for help*. Aggressive ventilation will result in gastric insufflation, with the consequent increased risk of regurgitation, as well as inhibiting the effectiveness of ventilation through diaphragmatic splinting (see Rule 51).
3 Raised airway pressure due to acute asthma, near-drowning, or in a newborn who has not taken an independent breath (especially common after Caesarian section). In these situations it is important to ensure that an adequate sized bag is used to provide the ventilation. The neonatal 240 ml bag is considered too small for this minority of neonates where the pressure generated is inadequate to expand the lungs. A minimal volume of 500 ml has been recommended to ensure that the inflation pressure is sustained for at least 0·5 seconds.[1] If the difficulty remains, the "pop off valve" can be held closed manually (some bags have a clip to allow this), or it can be exchanged for an adult valve.

The exceptions

A well trained and well practised resuscitation team is less likely to panic when presented with a child requiring ventilatory support (see Rule 1).

[1] Zideman D, Bingham R, Beattie T, *et al*. Recommendations on resuscitation of babies at birth. *Resuscitation* 1998;37:103–10.

The stomach will fill with air at the expense of the lungs

The reason

Air or oxygen delivered during resuscitation will follow the pathway of least resistance. This may be to the stomach. Positive pressure ventilation is particularly likely to lead to gastric distension because of the reduced pulmonary compliance and reduced oesophageal sphincter tone which accompany cardiorespiratory arrest.[1]

A small child's ribs join the sternum almost vertically, as opposed to adults where the ribs join perpendicularly. This means that there is little chest excursion during inspiration and the predominant method of ventilation is with the diaphragm. Gastric insufflation will inhibit ventilation in children by splinting the diaphragm. This may be relieved by gastric decompression with a nasogastric or orogastric tube.[1]

The exceptions

Gastric insufflation will not occur in a child who has an endotracheal tube or laryngeal mask airway *in situ* (see Rule 12). However, if a period of mouth-to-mouth/mask or bag-valve-mask ventilation has taken place prior to intubation, then gastric decompression is recommended to optimise ventilation.

[1] Berg M, Idris A, Berg R. Severe ventilatory compromise due to gastric distension during pediatric cardiopulmonary resuscitation. *Resuscitation* 1998;**36**:71–3.

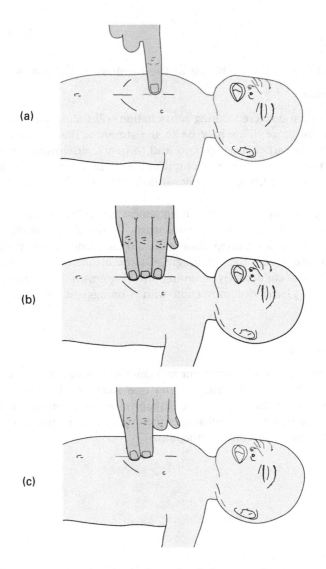

Chest compression technique for infants and neonates.

(a) Place your index finger on the inter-nipple line
(b) Place your middle and ring fingers adjacent to your index
    finger
(c) Lift up the index finger and apply compressions; you will
    always have the correct landmark – one finger's breadth
    below the inter-nipple line

Compression is one third of the chest diameter, irrespective of age

The reason

The technique of chest compression in children and infants has assigned specific values for the compression depth of, for example, "1·5–2·5 cm". While this is difficult to remember in theory, it is more difficult to achieve objectively in practice. A simple and rational alternative has been to introduce the concept of compressing to a depth of one third the total vertical height of the chest, measured from the firm surface on which the child is lying.

The compression rate has also been standardised to 100/minute, with one ventilation after every *five* compressions.

The exceptions

There is no exception to the rule for depth of compression.

In neonates the recommended compression rate is 120/minute, with one ventilation after every *three* compressions.[1] This can be achieved by remembering the following:

Say:
"A thousand-and-one, a thousand-and-puff, a thousand-and-one, a thousand-and-puff..."
Do:

| C | C | C | V | C | C | C | V |

where C = one compression and V = one ventilation

---

[1] Zideman D, Bingham R, Beattie T, *et al.* Recommendations on resuscitation of babies at birth. *Resuscitation* 1998;**37**:103–10.

CRT 2 is good for you

The reason

The capillary refill test (CRT) is an assessment of peripheral perfusion. It was first suggested as a simple method of grading shock by Beecher in 1947. He produced the following classification:

Capillary refill	Shock (grade)
Normal	None
Definite slowing	Slight to moderate
Very sluggish	Severe

Pressure is applied to a capillary bed for 5 seconds, firm enough to produce blanching. On release of pressure the capillary bed should become pink within 2 seconds. The fingernail, heel, or forehead may be used, but whichever is chosen the capillary bed should be above the level of the heart. In children, the most consistent results are achieved when the forehead is used.[1]

The exceptions

The capillary refill test has been criticised as an assessment of circulation in pre-hospital care, as peripheral perfusion is commonly reduced in the cold, irrespective of whether there is hypovolaemia.[2] In an assessment of over 300 normal individuals there was a significant reduction in the ability to assess CRT in the dark.[3] It has also been noted that there is significant observer variation, even between experienced observers, limiting its use in the assessment of ill or injured children.[4] These reservations apart, a **normal** CRT may still be an important indicator of an adequate circulation.

[1] Strozik K, Pieper C, Roller J. Capillary refill time in newborn babies: normal values. *Arch Dis Child* 1997;**76**:193–6.
[2] Schriger D, Baraff L. Defining normal capillary refill: variation with age, sex, and temperature. *Ann Emerg Med* 1988;**17**:932–5.
[3] Brown L, Prasad N, Whitley T. Adverse lighting condition effects on the assessment of capillary refill. *Am J Emerg Med* 1994;**12**:46–7.
[4] Gorelick M, Shaw K, Baker D. Effect of ambient temperature on capillary refill in healthy children. *Pediatrics* 1993;**92**:699–702.

You can get vascular access if you want it badly enough

The reason

Peripheral venous access can be difficult to obtain in children because the child will not cooperate with a painful procedure, or the paramedic or doctor is less practised in obtaining venous access in children than in adults.

When peripheral venous access fails the following routes should be considered:

- Intraosseous (see Rule 55)
- Percutaneous femoral vein access
- Cut down
- Central venous access.

The femoral vein can be accessed directly with a cannula-over-needle, or using the Seldinger technique. A cut down is most easily performed onto the long saphenous vein just above and anterior to the medial malleolus. Here the vein is superficial, the anatomy is consistent, and it is unlikely that any other local structure will be damaged during the procedure. Alternative sites include the sapheno-femoral junction in the groin, and the antecubital fossa veins (basilic and cephalic veins). Central venous access can be obtained via the internal jugular, or subclavian veins.

The exceptions

The child in whom none of these techniques is successful defies imagination. The intraosseous route in particular offers the simplest, most rapid, and effective alternative to peripheral venous access.

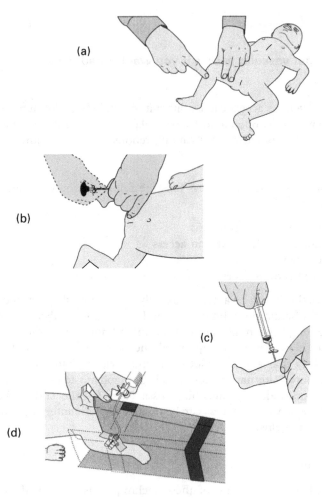

Inserting an intraosseous needle.

(a) Identify the landmarks (here showing just below and just medial to the tibial tuberosity)

(b) Insert the needle and trocar at 90° to the skin (you may aim slightly away fom the growth plate, but there is increased work of insertion through a greater bone distance)

(c) Check the position by aspiration of bone marrow, and by absence of resistance to a 5 ml flush

(d) Attach to a short connection tube and protect in a box splint (both of which help avoid inadvertent displacement of the needle)

IO it to him to get the drugs in

The reason

Attempts at peripheral venous access frequently fail in children (and adults), particularly when performed by inexperienced staff. This may lead to unacceptable delays in transport in the pre-hospital environment, or to delays in treatment in the emergency department.[1,2] In situations where peripheral intravenous access is difficult, or immediate effective venous access is imperative (for example, paediatric cardiac arrest or meningococcal septicaemia), then the intraosseous route should be used.

Intraosseal infusions were first described in 1922 by Drinker.[3] It was introduced as a clinical technique by Tocantis in 1941,[4,5] and was practised in Great Britain and South America as an emergency infusion route in the 1940s.[6] It is a suitable route for premature babies, term neonates, infants, children, and adults. The highest rates of success have been demonstrated in children under 3 years (85%), and the lowest rates in children over 10 years and in adults (in 50% the main failures were incorrect landmarks, or bending of needles).[7,8] Any drug and any fluid can be given by the intraosseous route, although infusion rates are slower than through a large peripheral vein.

The traditional site is just below and medial to the tibial tuberosity, but alternatives include the distal lateral femur, proximal lateral humerus, sternum, and clavicle. In adults, where the bone marrow cavity is relatively smaller, the preferred site is just above the medial malleolus. Intraosseous needles may be driven through the cortex either by manual force, or by using a corkscrew-type device, or by

[1] Jacobs L, Panic S. Pre-hospital care: what works, what does not. *Adv Trauma Crit Care* 1994;9:1.
[2] Orlowski J. Emergency alternatives to intravenous access. *Pediatr Clin North Am* 1994; 41:1183.
[3] Drinker C, Drinker K, Lund C. The circulation in the mammalian bone marrow. *Am J Physiol* 1922;62:1.
[4] Tocantis L, O'Neill J. Infusions of blood and other fluids into the general circulation via the bone marrow: technique and results. *Surg Gynecol Obstet* 1941;73:281.
[5] Tocantis L, O'Neill J, Jones H. Infusions of blood and other fluids via the bone marrow: application in pediatrics. *JAMA* 1941;117:1229.
[6] Bailey H. Cannulation of the sternum. *BMJ* 1946;1:661.
[7] Waisman M, Waisman D. Bone marrow infusion in adults. *J Trauma* 1997;42:288–93.
[8] Glaeser P, Hellmich T, Szewczuga D, *et al.* Five-year experience in prehospital intraosseous infusions in children and adults. *Ann Emerg Med* 1993;22:1119.

using a proprietary gun. Universal success has been claimed in a series of 50 adults, age range 27–78 years, when using the automatic bone injection gun.[7] Discomfort was said to be limited in the conscious adult group if 2–5 ml of bone marrow was aspirated and 2–5 ml of 1% lignocaine injected over 60 seconds, before starting any infusion.

The exceptions

A fracture in the chosen long bone is a contraindication to inserting an intraosseous needle: fluid will leak out from the fracture site and result in a compartment syndrome. A failed intraosseous needle insertion is a contraindication for the same reason. An intraosseous needle should not be inserted through localised infection.

Recognised complications are fracture, compartment syndrome (may also result from incomplete insertion), osteomyelitis, and fat embolism.

All sick children are hypoglycaemic
or . . . .
Follow ABC, but Don't Ever Forget Glucose!

The reason

Children have small reserves of glycogen that are rapidly depleted during serious illness or injury. Hypoglycaemia is therefore a common associated feature of any serious pathology. Importantly, it is a readily reversible cause of reduced level of response (with consequent threat to the airway) and convulsions. A capillary blood sugar should be tested as part of the primary survey in all emergency situations involving children.

Glucose is replaced as a 10% solution (2–5 ml/kg)[1] rather than the concentrated 50% solution used in adults. This avoids wide swings in osmotic pressure that may result in cerebral oedema, which can be fatal.[1-3]

The exceptions

Diabetic ketoacidosis is a serious illness characterised by a raised blood glucose concentration. An elevated blood glucose is reported as an idiosyncratic feature of subarachnoid haemorrhage. An excess of endogenous or exogenous steroids may also result in hyperglycaemia.

[1] Jewkes F. Paediatric advanced life support. *Pre-hospital Immediate Care* 1998;2:83–9.
[2] Advanced Life Support Group. *Advanced Paediatric Life Support*, 2nd edn. London: BMJ Publishing, 1997.
[3] Shah A, Stanhope R, Mathew D. Hazards of pharmacological tests of growth hormone secretion in childhood. *BMJ* 1992;304:173–4.

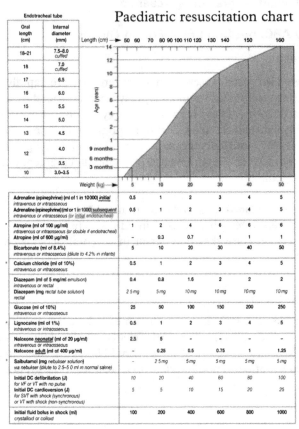

Paediatric resuscitation chart

Endotracheal tube

Oral length (cm)	Internal diameter (mm)
18–21	7.5–8.0 cuffed
18	7.0 cuffed
17	6.5
16	6.0
15	5.5
14	5.0
13	4.5
12	4.0
	3.5
10	3.0–3.5

Length (cm) → 50 60 70 80 90 100 110 120 130 140 150 160

Age (years)

9 months, 6 months, 3 months

Weight (kg) →

	5	10	20	30	40	50
Adrenaline (epinephrine) (ml of 1 in 10000) *initial* intravenous or intraosseous	0.5	1	2	3	4	5
Adrenaline (epinephrine) (ml of 1 in 1000) subsequent intravenous or intraosseous (or initial endotracheal)	0.5	1	2	3	4	5
Atropine (ml of 100 µg/ml) intravenous or intraosseous (or double if endotracheal)	1	2	4	6	6	6
Atropine (ml of 600 µg/ml)	–	0.3	0.7	1	1	1
Bicarbonate (ml of 8.4%) intravenous or intraosseous (dilute to 4.2% in infants)	5	10	20	30	40	50
Calcium chloride (ml of 10%) intravenous or intraosseous	0.5	1	2	3	4	5
Diazepam (ml of 5 mg/ml emulsion) intravenous or rectal	0.4	0.8	1.6	2	2	2
Diazepam (mg rectal tube solution) rectal	2.5 mg	5 mg	10 mg	10 mg	10 mg	10 mg
Glucose (ml of 10%) intravenous or intraosseous	25	50	100	150	200	250
Lignocaine (ml of 1%) intravenous or intraosseous	0.5	1	2	3	4	5
Naloxone *neonatal* (ml of 20 µg/ml) intravenous or intraosseous	2.5	5	–	–	–	–
Naloxone adult (ml of 400 µg/ml)	–	0.25	0.5	0.75	1	1.25
Salbutamol (mg nebuliser solution) via nebuliser (dilute to 2.5–5.0 ml in normal saline)	–	2.5 mg	5 mg	5 mg	5 mg	5 mg
Initial DC defibrillation (J) for VF or VT with no pulse	10	20	40	60	80	100
Initial DC cardioversion (J) for SVT with shock (synchronous) or VT with shock (non-synchronous)	5	5	10	15	20	25
Initial fluid bolus in shock (ml) crystalloid or colloid	100	200	400	600	800	1000

* **CAUTION!** Non-standard drug concentrations may be available.
Use **Atropine** 100 µg/ml or prepare by diluting 1 mg to 10 ml or 600 µg to 6 ml in normal saline
Note that 1 ml of **calcium chloride** 10% is equivalent to 3 ml of **calcium gluconate** 10%.
Use **Lignocaine** (without adrenaline) 1% or give twice the volume of 0.5% or dilute appropriately.
Salbutamol may also be given by slow intravenous injection (4–6 µg/kg), but beware of the different concentrations available (eg 50 and 500 µg/ml).

The revised Oakley chart.
(Reproduced with permission from the author.)

To get the dose of adrenaline (epinephrine), work out the weight and divide by ten

The reason

The doses of drugs used in paediatric resuscitation are calculated from the child's weight, or an estimation of the weight.

The initial dose of adrenaline (epinephrine) for all cardiac arrest rhythms is 10 micrograms/kg (0·01 mg/kg). This is equivalent to 0·1 ml/kg of 1:10 000 adrenaline (epinephrine) solution. If, for example, the child weighs 15 kg the correct dose is 1.5 ml of 1:10 000 adrenaline (epinephrine) (or 150 micrograms).

This raises the question, "How do you work out the weight of a child?" There are three principal methods:

1 Weigh the child (but this is impractical in a critical situation). Ask a parent (but in the UK, the answer will often be in stones and pounds, rather than in kilograms).
2 Relate the length of the child to its weight (this can be read from an Oakley chart[1,2] – a paediatric resuscitation chart, or a Broselow tape[3,4] – a proprietary tape that is laid next to the child, and where the heel touches there is a box of drug doses and invasive equipment sizes for that weight of child).
3 Use a formula (accurate from 1–10 years):

$$Weight\ (kg) = [age\ in\ years + 4] \times 2$$

The exceptions

The second and any subsequent doses of adrenaline (epinephrine) are 100 micrograms/kg (0·1 mg/kg). For simplicity, the same volume can be administered if the rescuer uses 1:1000 solution.

[1] Oakley P. Inaccuracy and delay in decision making in paediatric resuscitation, and a proposed reference chart to reduce error. *BMJ* 1988;**297**:817–9.
[2] Oakley P, Phillips B, Molyneux E, Mackway-Jones K. *BMJ* 1993;**306**:1096–8.
[3] Luten R, Wears R, Broselow J, *et al.* Length-based endotracheal tube and emergency equipment in pediatrics. *Ann Emerg Med* 1992;**21**:900–4.
[4] Reyes T, Childs P. The Broselow Paediatric Resuscitation Book: a guide to drugs and equipment. Brighton: Vital Signs Ltd, 1994.

Penicillin V halves mortality

The reason

Neisseria meningitidis is an important cause of bacterial meningitis in infants and young children, with a second peak of incidence in teenagers and young adults. Its relative importance has grown following the reduction in *Haemophilus influenzae* invasive infections with the introduction of the Hib vaccine in 1990. Meningococcal meningitis and meningococcal septicaemia constitute the spectrum of "meningococcal disease". There is a predominantly septicaemic illness in about one fifth of cases. The overall mortality of meningococcal disease is around 8% (up to 5% in meningitis, rising to 15–20% with septicaemia) and this is improved by the early administration of antibiotics.[1-3] The infection is characteristically fulminant, with rapid clinical deterioration and death in a matter of hours. The mortality is particularly high in meningococcal septicaemia when there has been a delay in diagnosis or treatment (up to 60% where there is septic shock).[3]

Current recommendations in England and Wales are for the attending general practitioner to administer intramuscular penicillin if the diagnosis is considered. Infants receive 300 mg, children 1–9 years receive 600 mg, and those 10 years or more receive 1200 mg.[1] The use of penicillin by general practitioners has been shown to reduce mortality by over 50% in those septicaemic patients presenting with signs of shock.[2]

The exceptions

Although benzylpenicillin has been the traditional antibiotic for *Neisseria meningitidis*, penicillin-resistant meningococci have been isolated in Spain, South Africa, and the UK.[4] The first line antimicrobial treatment in hospital is therefore a third generation

[1] Calman K. Meningococcal infection: meningitis and septicaemia. London: Department of Health PL/CMO(94)2, 1994.
[2] Cartwright K, Reilly S, White D, Stuart J. Early treatment with parenteral penicillin in meningococcal disease. *BMJ* 1992;305:143–52.
[3] PHLS Meningococcal Infections Working Group. Control of meningococcal disease: guidance for consultants in communicable disease control. *CDR Rev* 1995;13:189–95.
[4] Klein N, Heyderman R, Levin M. Antibiotic choices for meningitis beyond the neonatal period. *Arch Dis Child* 1992;67:157–61.

cephalosporin (cefotaxime 200 mg/kg/day in three or four divided doses, or ceftriaxone 80 mg/kg/day in a single dose).[5] Additional penicillin is not needed – although it is often still given if omitted pre-hospital.[6,7] The analogy is that there is nothing to be gained from putting ordinary unleaded petrol on top of super plus unleaded!

For meningitis and septicaemia in infants 1–3 months old additional ampicillin 200 mg/kg/day is recommended, to ensure activity against an increased spectrum of organisms that includes *Escherichia coli*, *Listeria monocytogenes* and salmonella species.[4,7–9]

[5] Hodgetts T, Brett A, Castle N. The early management of meningococcal disease. *J Accid Emerg Med* 1998;15:72–6.
[6] Nadel S, Habibi P, Levin M. Management of meningococcal septicaemia. *Care of the Critically Ill* 1995;11:33–8.
[7] Levin M, Heyderman R. Bacterial meningitis. In: *Recent advances in paediatrics, No 9*. Edinburgh: Churchill Livingstone, 1991.
[8] Bégué R, Steele R. Ceftriaxone in pediatrics: severe infections. *Rev Contemp Pharmacother* 1995;6:401–13.
[9] Prober C. Infections of the central nervous system. In: Nelson W (ed). *Textbook of Pediatrics*, 15th edn. Philadelphia: WB Saunders, 1996.

Rule 59

Parents are part of the resuscitation team

The reason

It has been established practice to exclude the relatives of the critically ill from witnessing their resuscitation, either in the accident and emergency (A&E) department, the intensive care unit, or on the ward. The rationale is that family members will be distressed by the event, and the performance of clinical staff will be compromised[1,2] – the reality being that the inexperienced doctor lacks confidence in his or her ability to manage the crisis.[3] In a study of 81 doctors and nurses working in A&E, nurses were generally in favour of the presence of relatives. Doctors were more likely to be in favour with increasing seniority.[3] Reasons for opposing this strategy were a belief that relatives would impede resuscitation (79%), a fear that the resuscitation would be seen as chaotic (49%), a fear that insensitive comments may be made by staff (43%), and a fear of increased litigation (20%). This study has been criticised for its small sample size and questionnaire bias, but the finding that nurses were in favour of the presence of relatives was consistent with results from five other centres.[4]

The presumption that relatives will be distressed is not supported by research. In a randomised controlled study of relatives' psychological response to inclusion or exclusion from the A&E resuscitation room, there was no evidence that those who witnessed the event were more distressed than the controls. Conversely, when assessed 3 months after the event there was a trend towards reduced symptoms of grief and less post-traumatic avoidance behaviour in the exposed group.[5]

The problem is compounded in paediatric resuscitation. A parent or guardian invariably accompanies a critically ill child. In such cases the parent can offer the child reassurance to facilitate the necessary invasive procedures, and provide important history to aid diagnosis

[1] Osuagwn C. ED codes: keep the family out. *J Emerg Nurs* 1991;17:36.
[2] Schilling R. No room for spectators. *BMJ* 1994;309:406.
[3] Mitchell M, Lynch M. Should relatives be allowed in the resuscitation room? *J Accid Emerg Med* 1997;14:366–9.
[4] Cooke M, Wilson S, Anthony A *et al.* Should relatives be allowed in the resuscitation room. *J Accid Emerg Med* 1998;15:364.
[5] Robinson S, Mackenzie-Ross S, Campbell Hewson G, Egleston C, Prevost A. Psychological effect of witnessed resuscitation on bereaved relatives. *Lancet* 1998;352: 614–7.

and plan treatment. An attempt to exclude parents is to deny these advantages, cause stress through separation, and, at worst, threaten the safety of staff in the most determined case.

Adults who collapse are often alone, or are not accompanied in the ambulance by their partner. The issue of a relative's presence in the resuscitation room during the immediate reception phase is therefore less frequent, although still important.

The exceptions

Palmer points out that the only way of preventing post-traumatic stress reactions or mental illness is by not exposing the individuals to traumatic events.[6] While this is true, it should be balanced with a careful exposure to the resuscitation to aid the grieving process.

The advocacy of witnessed resuscitation is currently restricted to the A&E department, where there is space to accommodate relatives, staff available to act as a chaperone, and continuity in the staff of the resuscitation team (particularly where the arrest is managed primarily by A&E medical staff). While there are clear similarities in available resources in areas such as the intensive care unit, it is much less likely on the general wards.

Careful consideration should be given to restricting access to parents of a critically ill child who is the subject of non-accidental injury.

---

[6] Palmer I. Should relatives be allowed in the resuscitation room? *J Accid Emerg Med* 1998;**15**:364.

Do not resuscitate the date of birth

The reason

The decision to start resuscitation of a child pre-hospital, or to continue resuscitation on arrival at hospital, is frequently one driven by emotion rather than a realistic opportunity for success.

Consider these two scenarios:

1   A 2-year-old girl who has been pyrexial and vomiting for several hours overnight, develops a widespread purpuric rash. The child stops breathing and is rushed by car to hospital without any basic life support. On arrival the child is in asystole.
2   A 79-year-old man with known ischaemic heart disease collapses in the general practitioner's surgery. Basic life support is provided immediately and the ambulance arrives with a defibrillator in 6 minutes. The man is found to be in ventricular fibrillation.

It is likely that the elderly patient has a better chance of survival. However, the desire for the resuscitation to be effective, perhaps reflected in the aggressiveness of the attempt, is likely to be greater for the child.

The exceptions

There are no logical exceptions to this rule.

Reader's rules

Use this space to make a note of your own rules. If you would like your ideas to be considered for a future edition of *Resuscitation Rules*, please send them to:

> BMJ Books
> BMA House
> Tavistock Square
> London WC1H 9JR

Or e-mail direct to the author at: tim.hodgetts@virgin.net

All contributions will be appropriately acknowledged.

Index